Getting Ready for My MRI Scan

An MRI Scan Book for Kids –   Preparation and Recovery

This book belongs to:

Written by Dr. Fei Zheng-Ward   Illustrated by Moch. Fajar Shobaru

Copyright © 2025 Fei Zheng-Ward

All rights reserved. Published by Fei Zheng-Ward, an imprint of FZWbooks. No part of this book may be copied, reproduced, recorded, transmitted, or stored by any means or in any form, electronic or mechanical, without obtaining prior written permission from the copyright owner.

Identifiers: ISBN 979-8-89318-131-9 (eBook)
              ISBN 979-8-89318-132-6 (paperback)
              ISBN 979-8-89318-133-3 (hardcover)

An MRI (Magnetic Resonance Imaging) is a big, donut-shaped camera machine that lets your doctor see inside your body, like your brain, arms, legs, and tummy.

*What does this machine remind you of?
A cave? A playground tunnel?
A new adventure?*

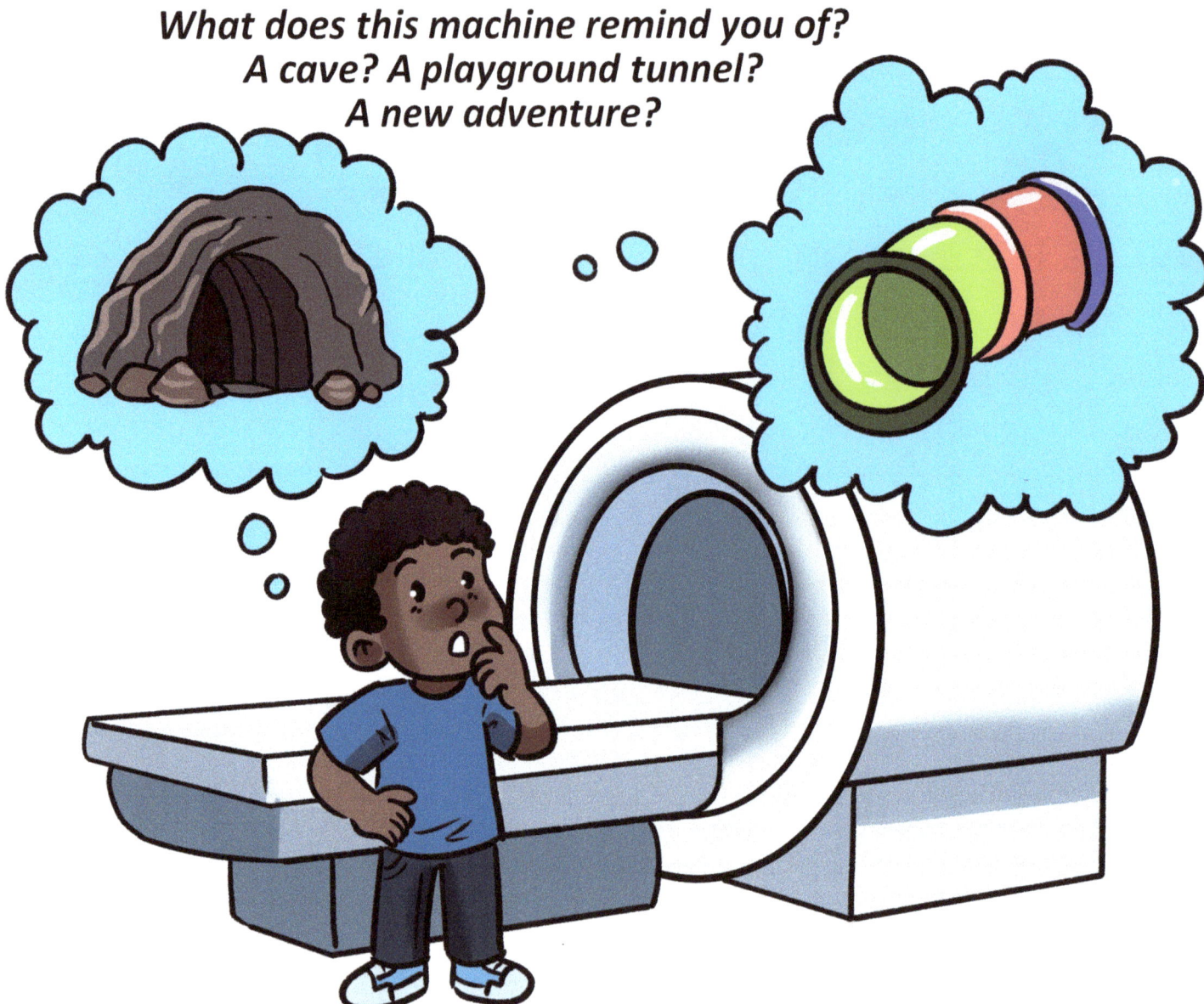

This special camera uses a big magnet and radio waves to make detailed pictures of your body.

The magnet and the radio waves won't hurt you.

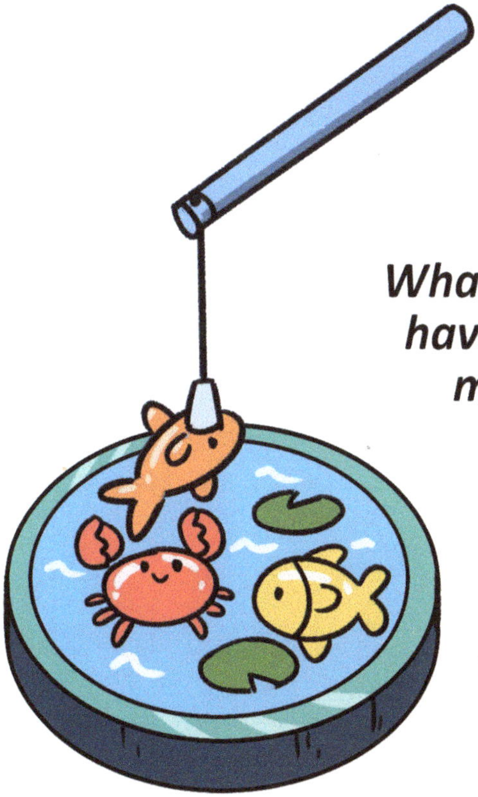

What toy do you have that uses magnets?

magnetic fishing game

magnetic building set

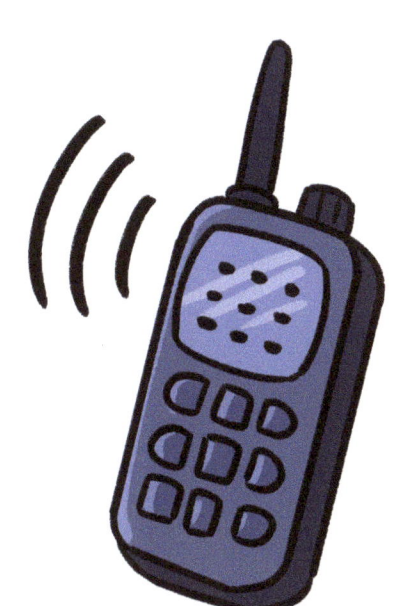

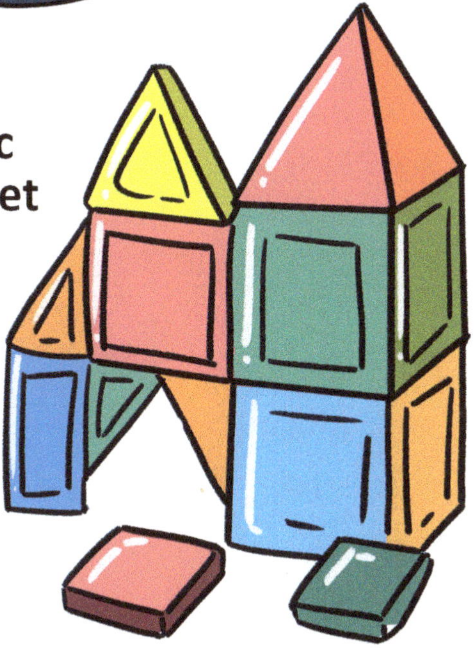

Radio waves are invisible energy waves that travel through the air.

The music you hear on the radio and the voices you hear on a walkie-talkie are both carried by radio waves.

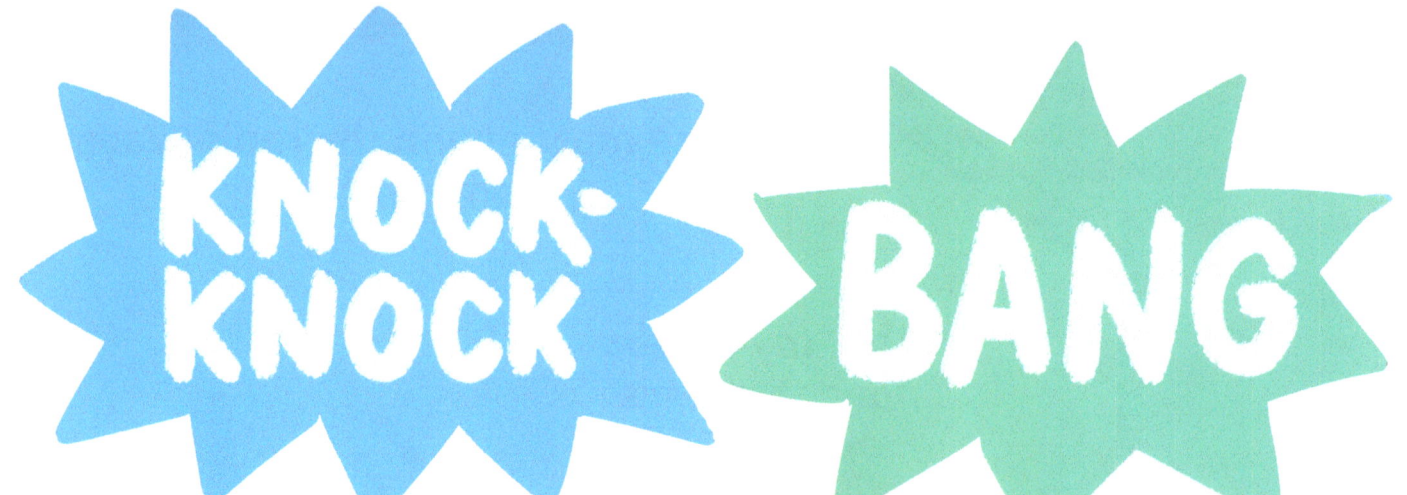
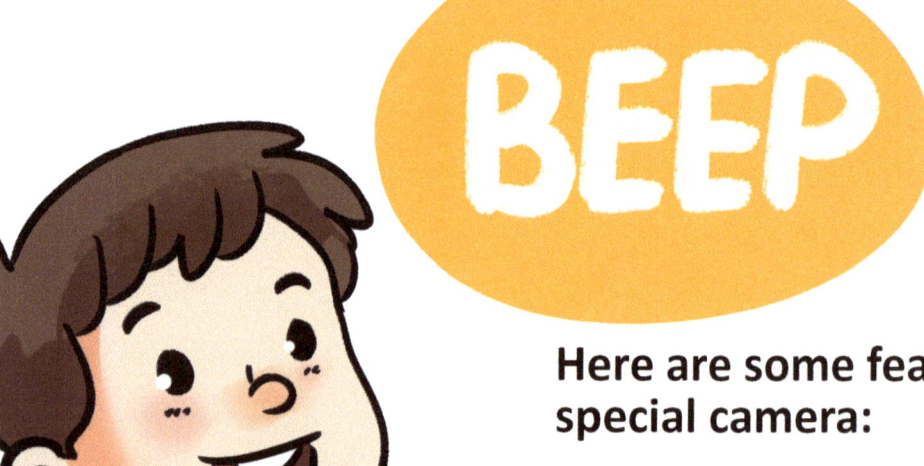

Here are some features of this special camera:

- It makes loud sounds such as "knock-knock," "bang," "beep," or buzzing noises
- For this camera to take great pictures, you'll need to stay very still
- While it takes pictures, you won't feel any pain

Think of this loud camera machine as a bunch of clumsy, silly robots cooking in the kitchen, dropping different pots and pans on the floor and making all the funny noises you hear.

You'll get earplugs to help block out the sound.

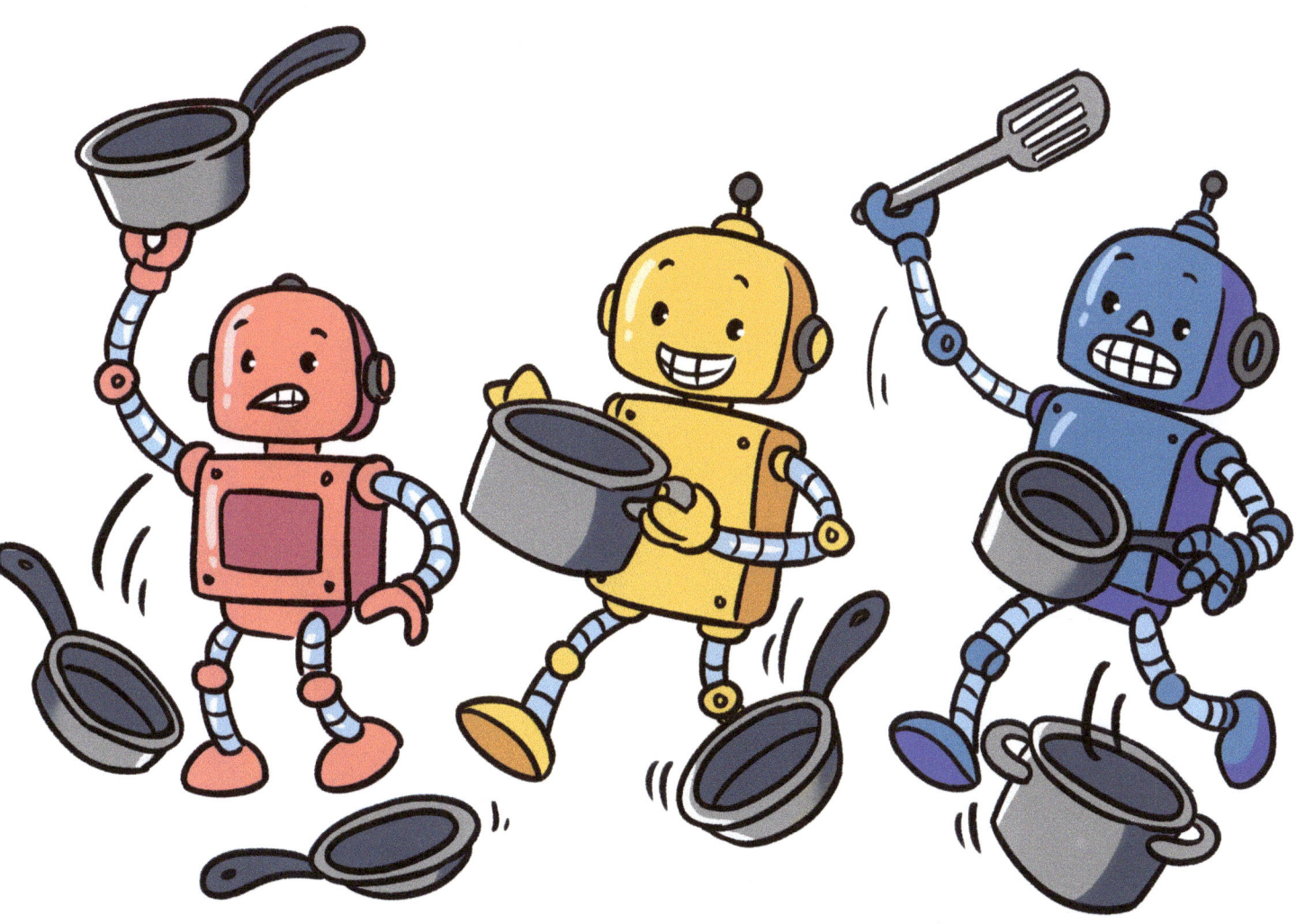

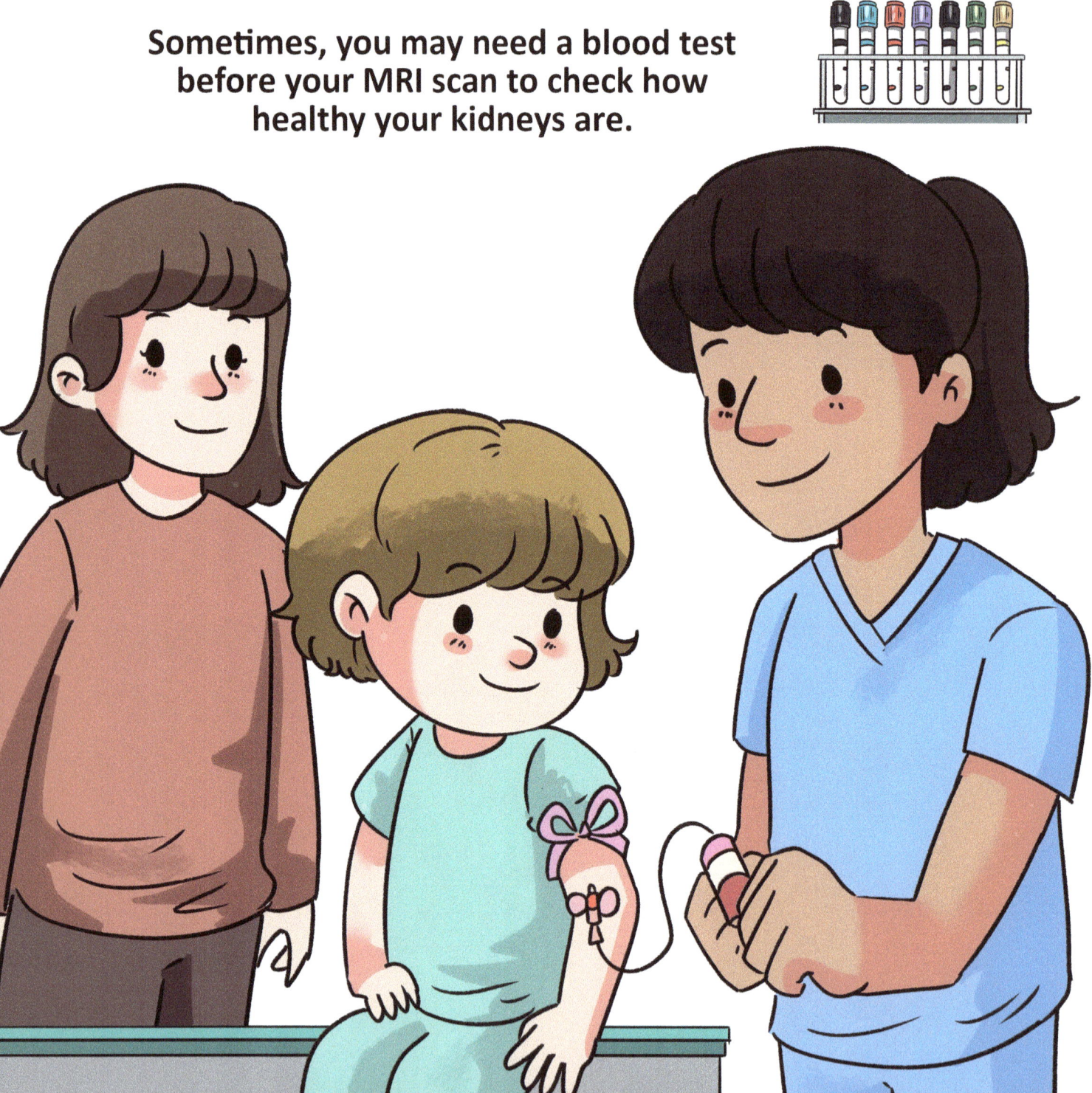
Sometimes, you may need a blood test before your MRI scan to check how healthy your kidneys are.

They will put a long and thick rubber band around your arm. Then, your skin is cleaned before they use a small needle to gently go under your skin and into the vein. It feels like a quick, small pinch.

Tip: With the rubber band around your arm, you can make your veins bigger and easier to see by making a fist a few times.

Fun Fact: Some needles look like butterflies.

They are needles with wings, and they come in different colors. If you get a needle with butterfly wings, circle the color below.

red   green   yellow   blue   pink   orange   purple

A little bit of your blood is collected into a small plastic tube. Once done, the needle is removed, and you get a bandage on that spot.

What do you want to do when they're drawing your blood?

____ watch   ____ hold onto my favorite toy

____ turn my head away   ____ hold my parent or guardian's hand

____ listen to music   ____ watch a short video

This is not easy, but you're brave and you can do this!

For your MRI scan, don't wear anything with metal, like sparkly jewelry, hairpins, or clips.

If you wear glasses, you will need to remove them before your scan.

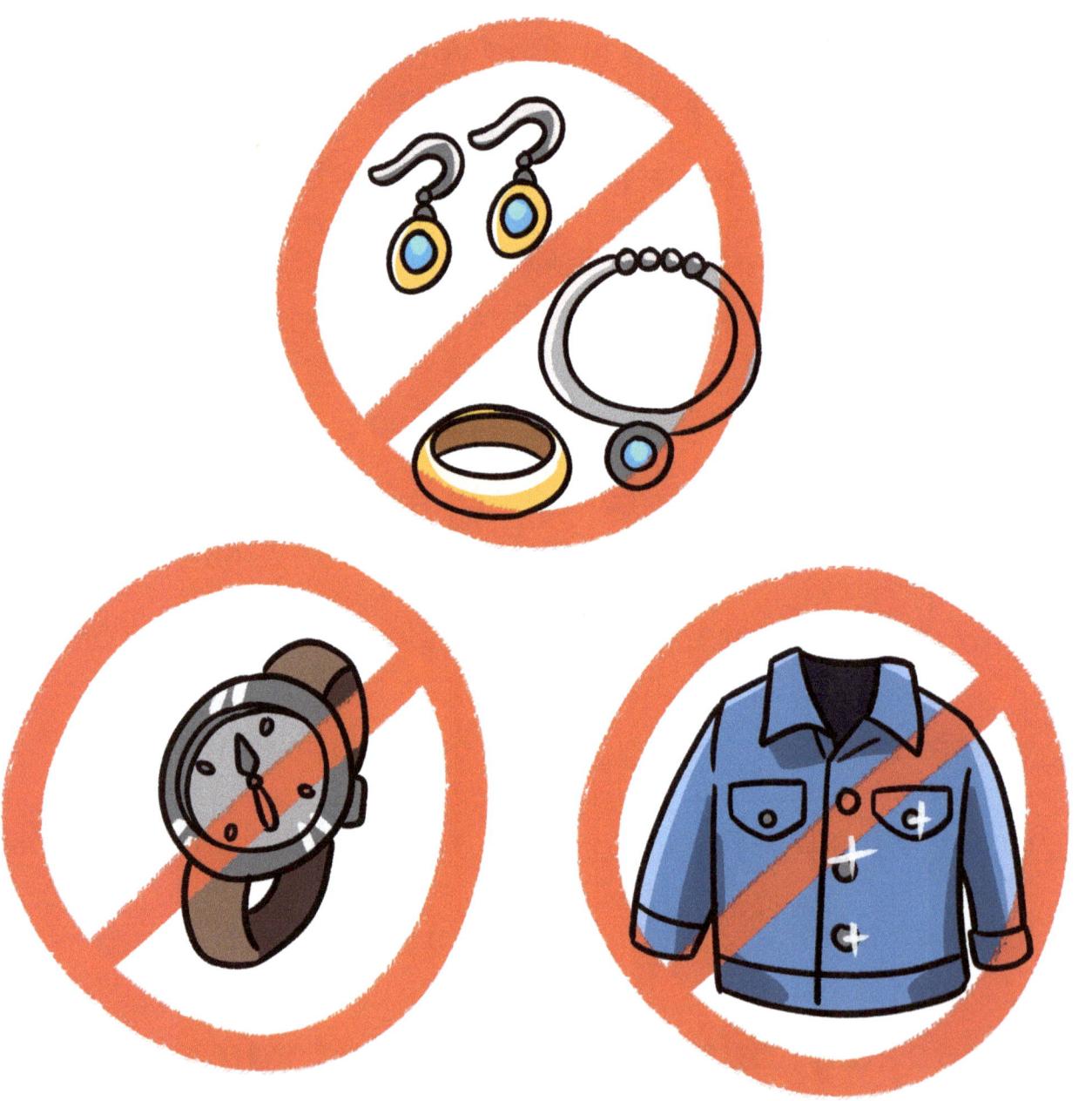

Don't worry, your grown-up will help you.

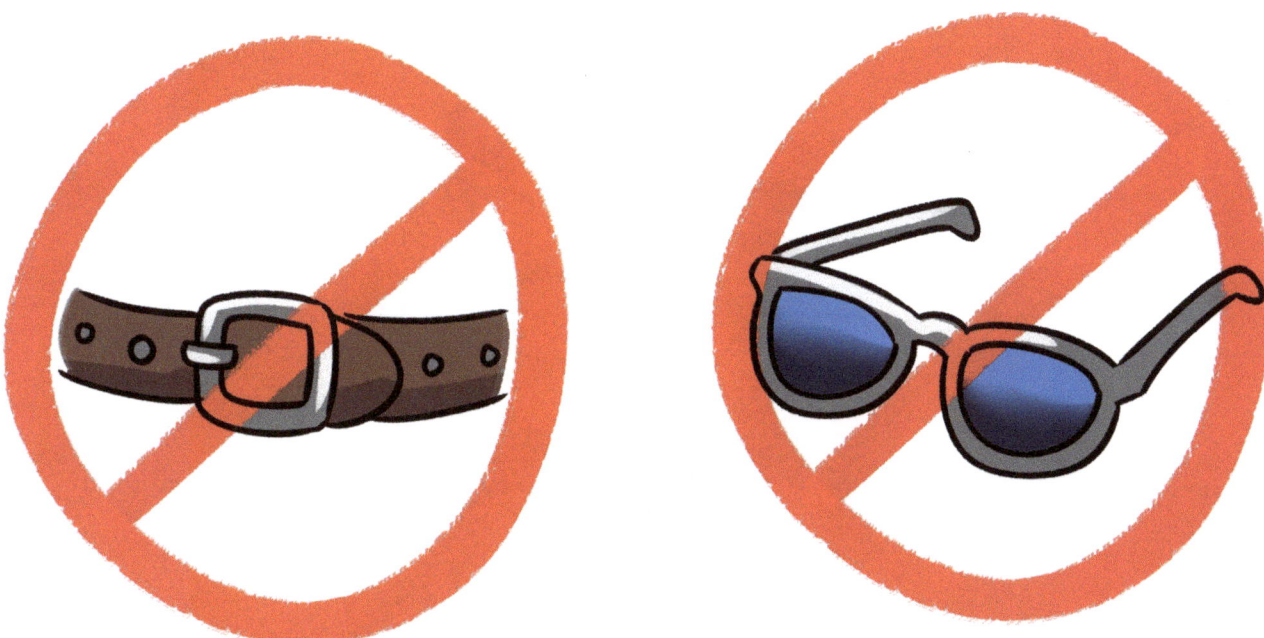

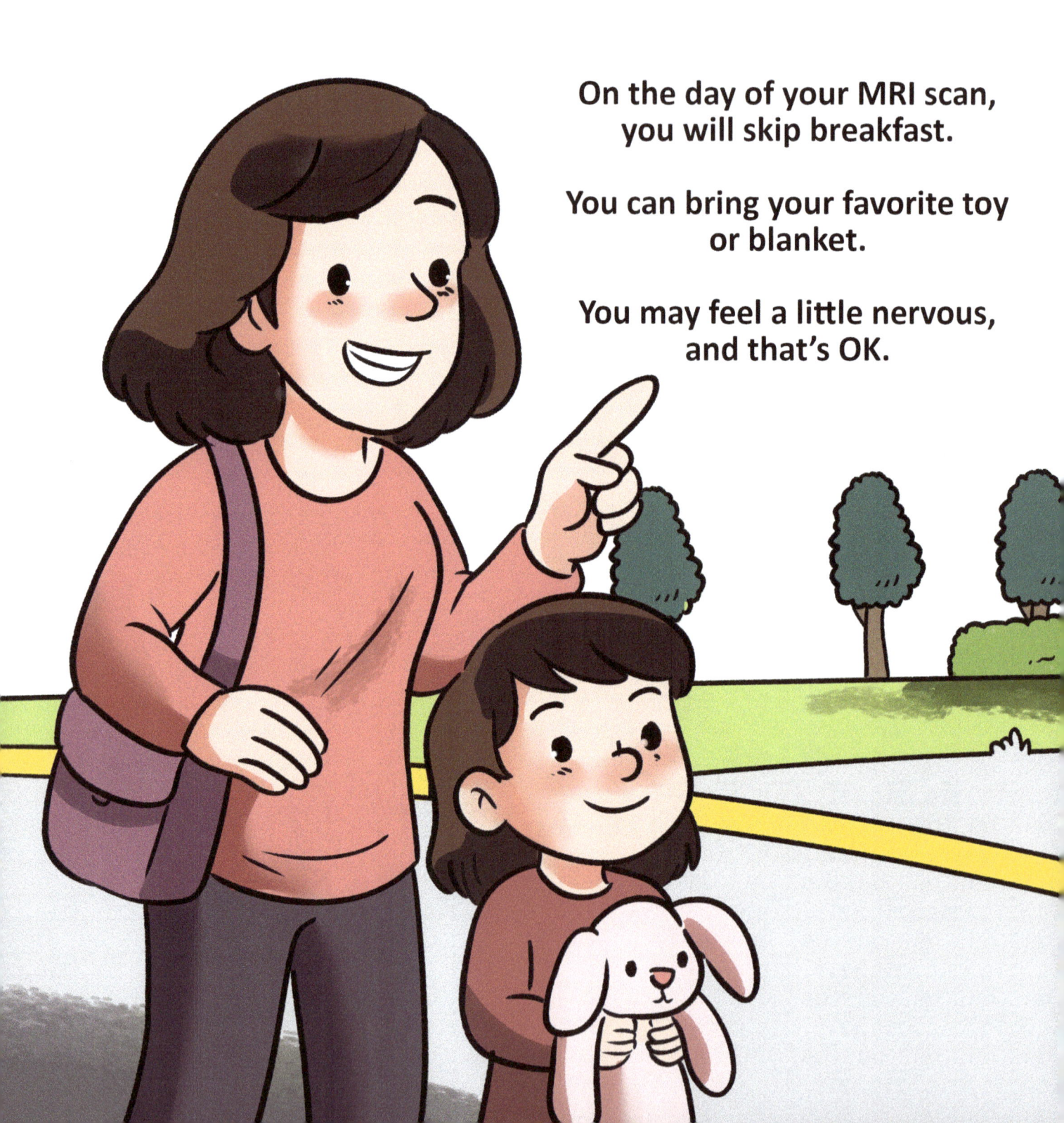

What do you plan to bring with you?

Check your answer below.

- ☐ Blanket
- ☐ Toy
- ☐ Book

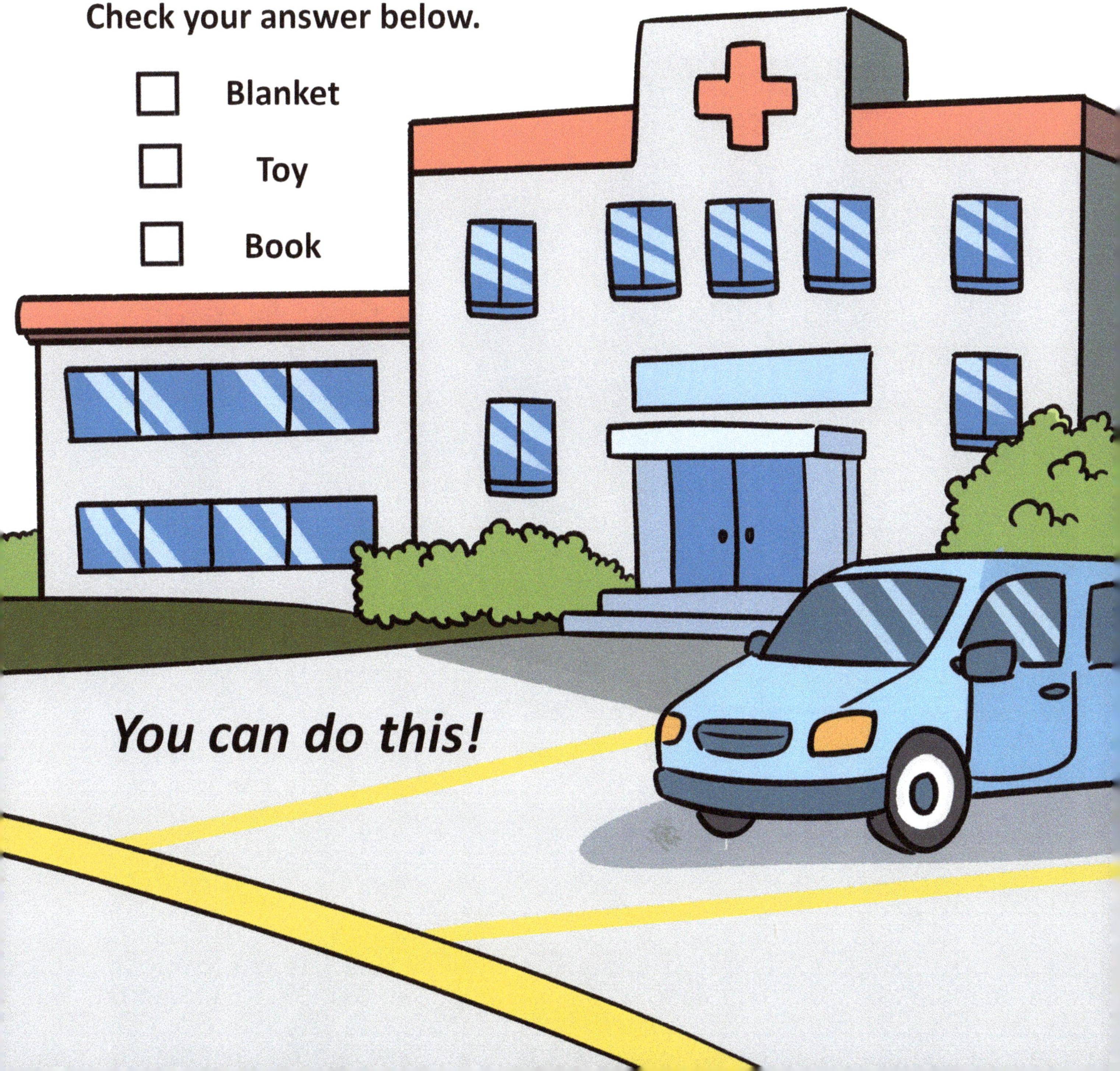

You can do this!

You will check in at the hospital and give them your name and birth date.

Then, you will receive a special wristband. Now everyone will know your name.

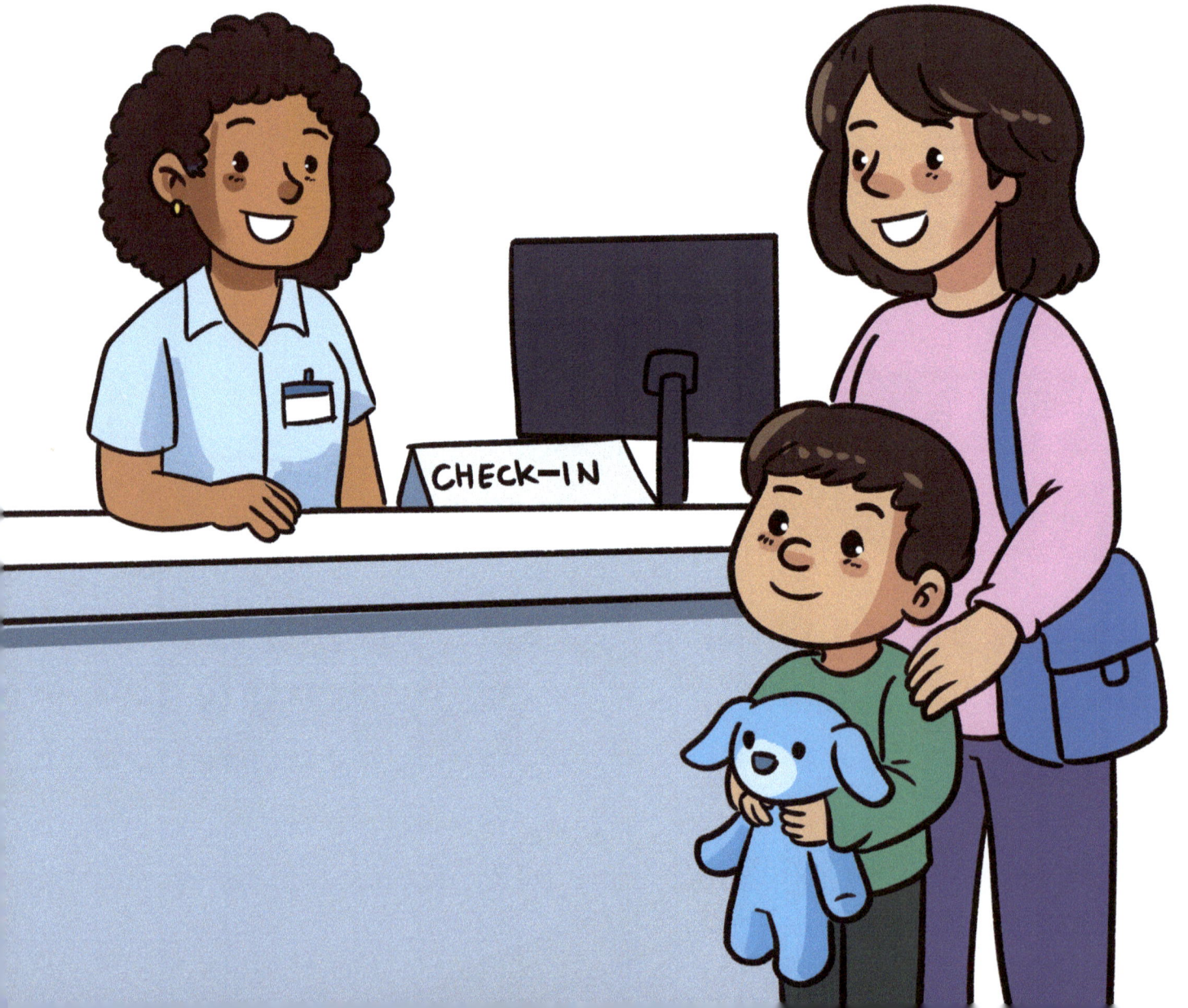

What color wristband will you get?
Circle the color of your wristband below.

Red   Green   Yellow   Blue   Pink   Orange

Purple   Black   White

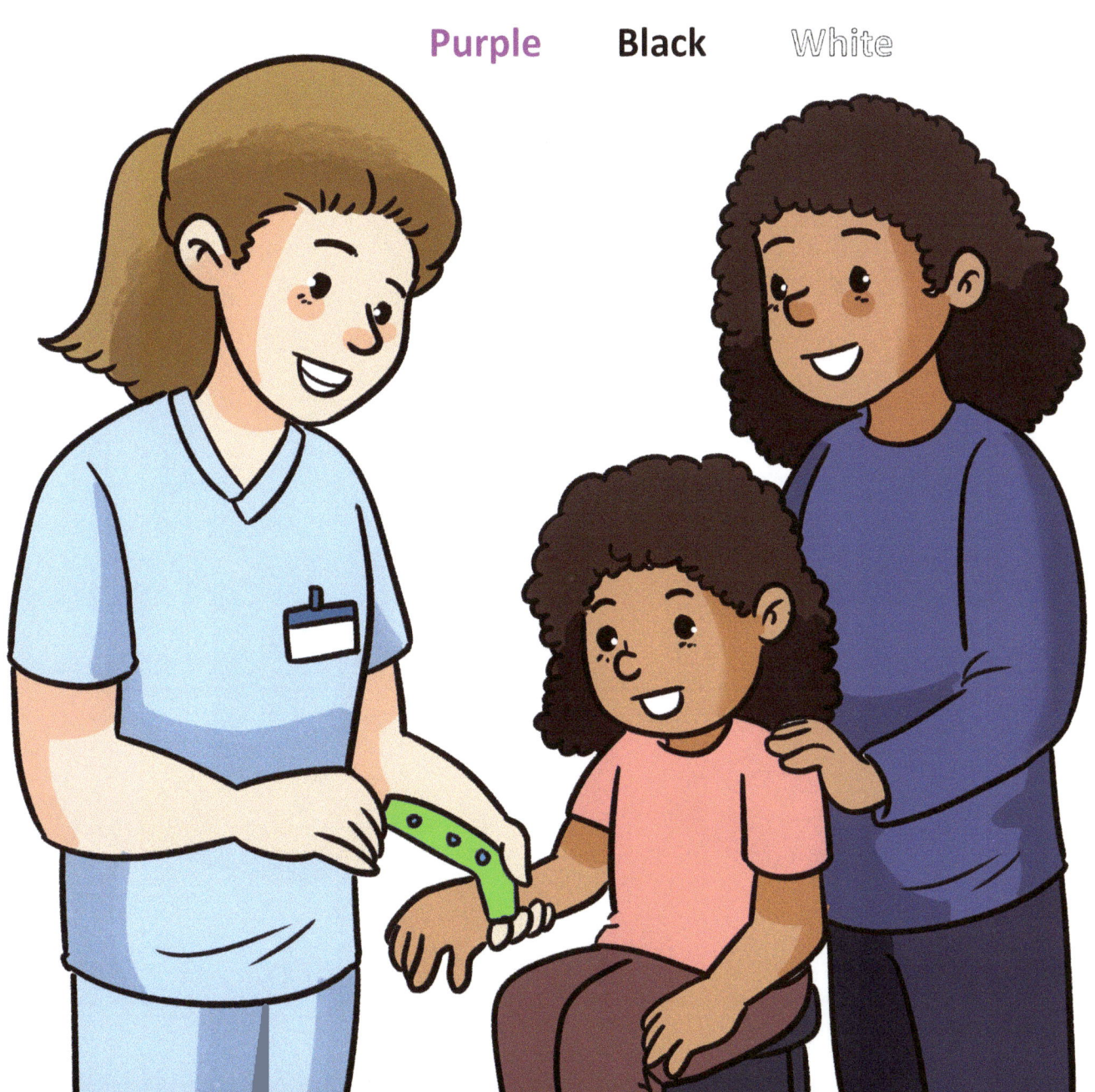

They will check your weight and height before getting you ready.

Do you know how much you weigh?

Do you know how tall you are?

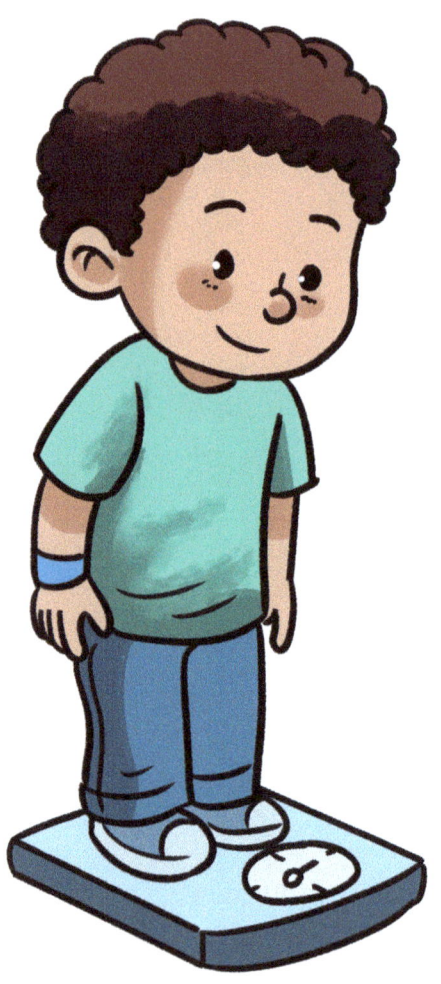

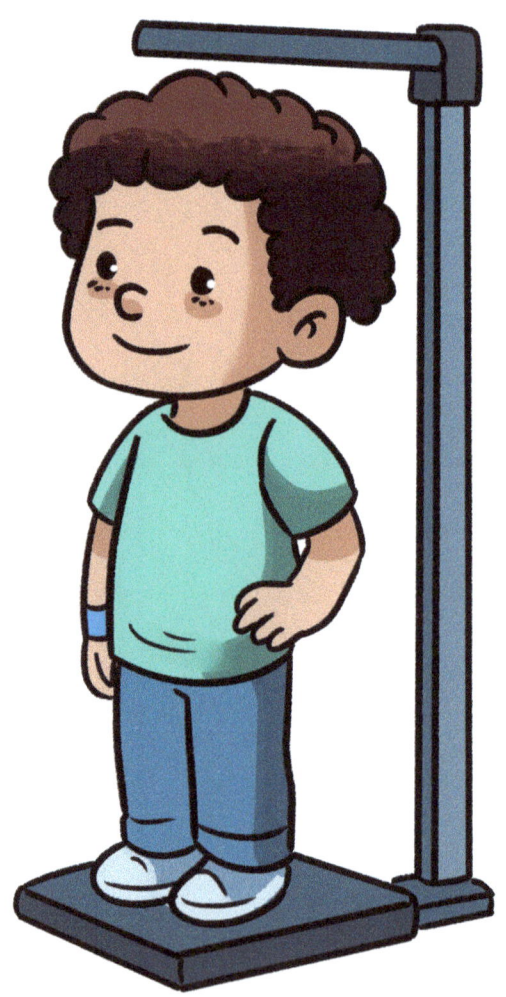

My weight is: _____

My height is: _____

You will change into a new outfit, put on a gown that looks like a backward superhero cape, and wear some cozy socks.

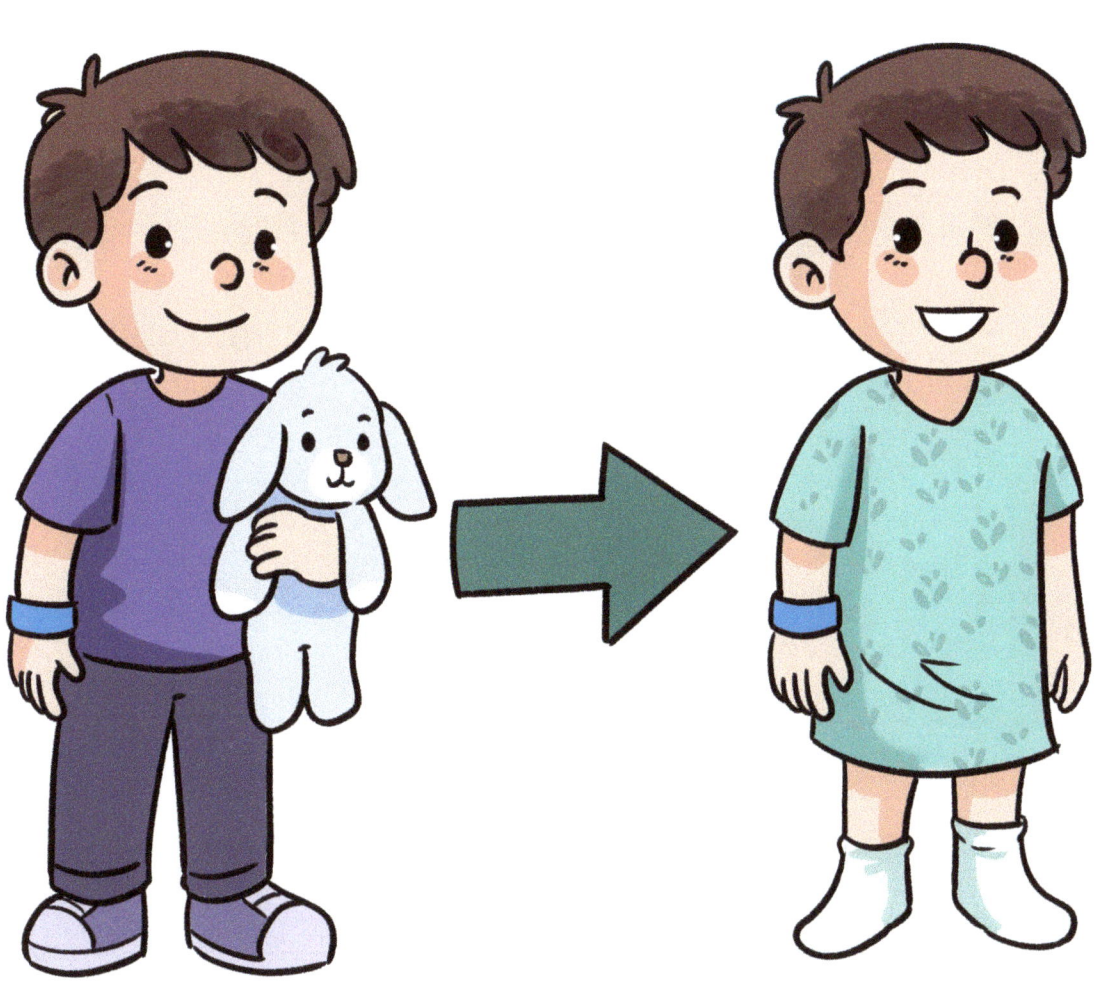

Your nurse may put a clip on your finger or toe to see how much oxygen is in your body.

Oxygen keeps your body working so you can do the things you love.

Which finger or toe do you want to use?

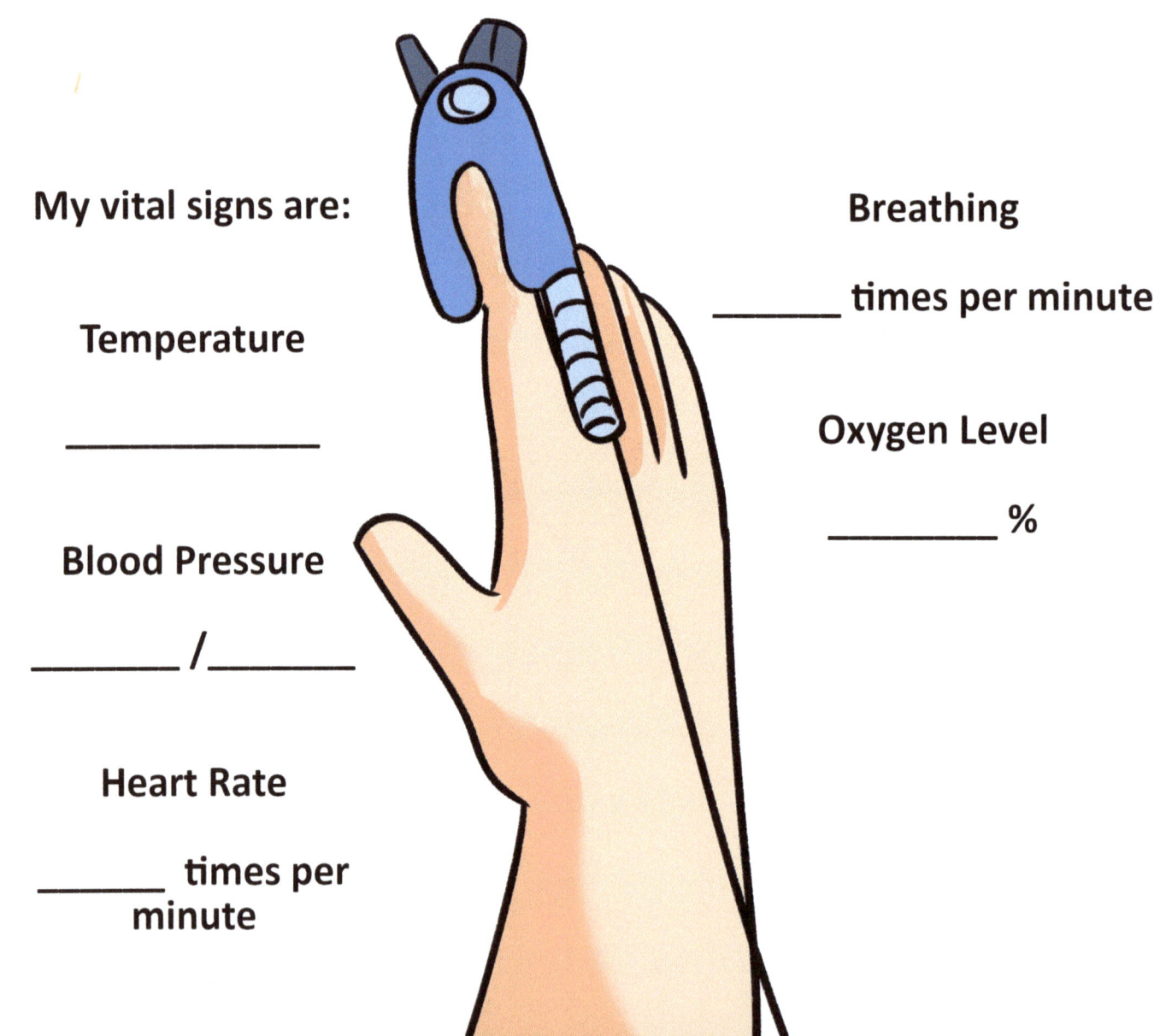

My vital signs are:

Temperature

_____

Blood Pressure

_____ / _____

Heart Rate

_____ times per minute

Breathing

_____ times per minute

Oxygen Level

_____ %

You'll get a blood pressure cuff around your arm or leg.
The cuff will give you a BIG hug.

Don't forget to stay still while they're examining you.

Are you ready?

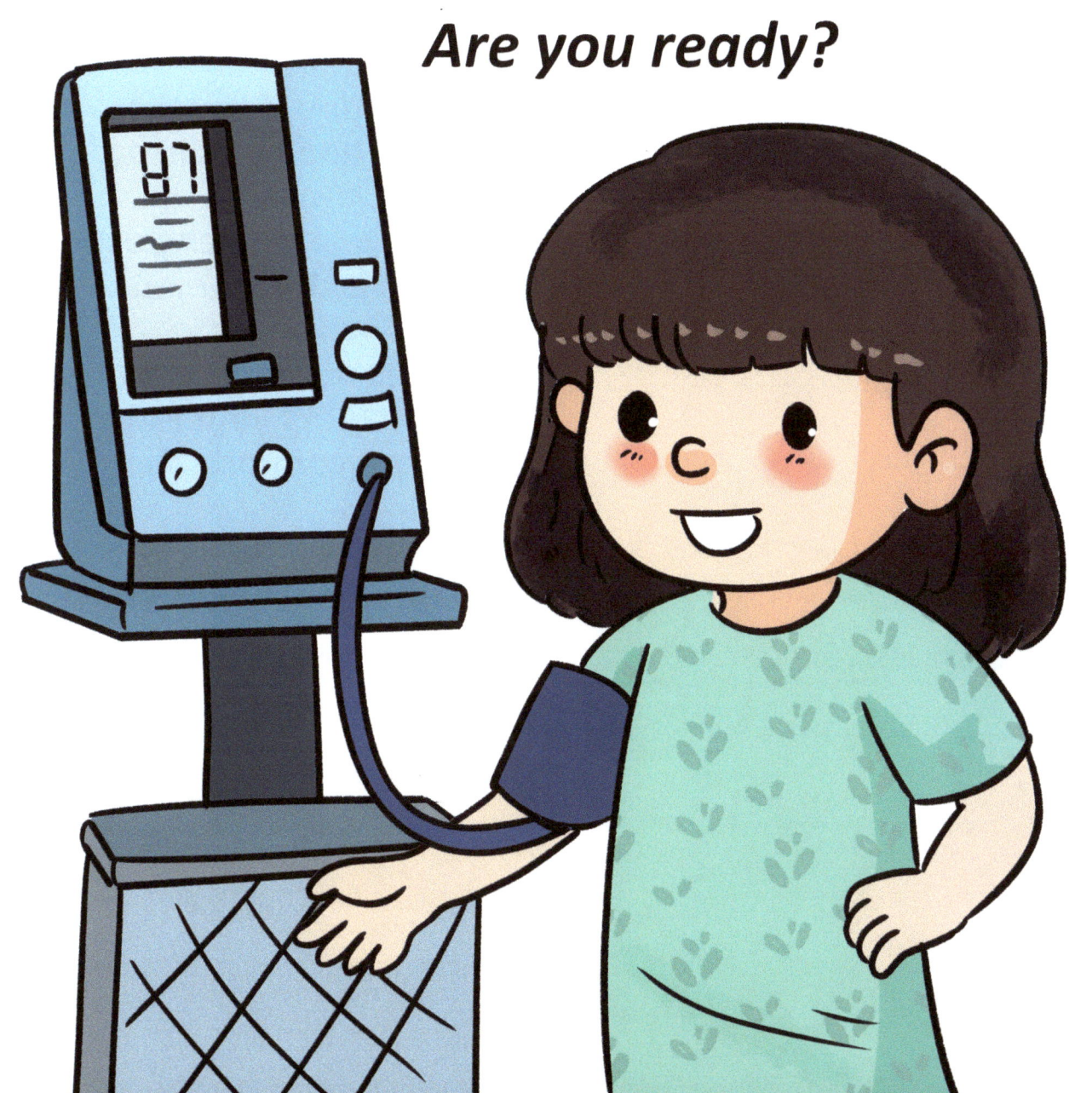

Sometimes, you may be given a sweet medicine to help you relax.

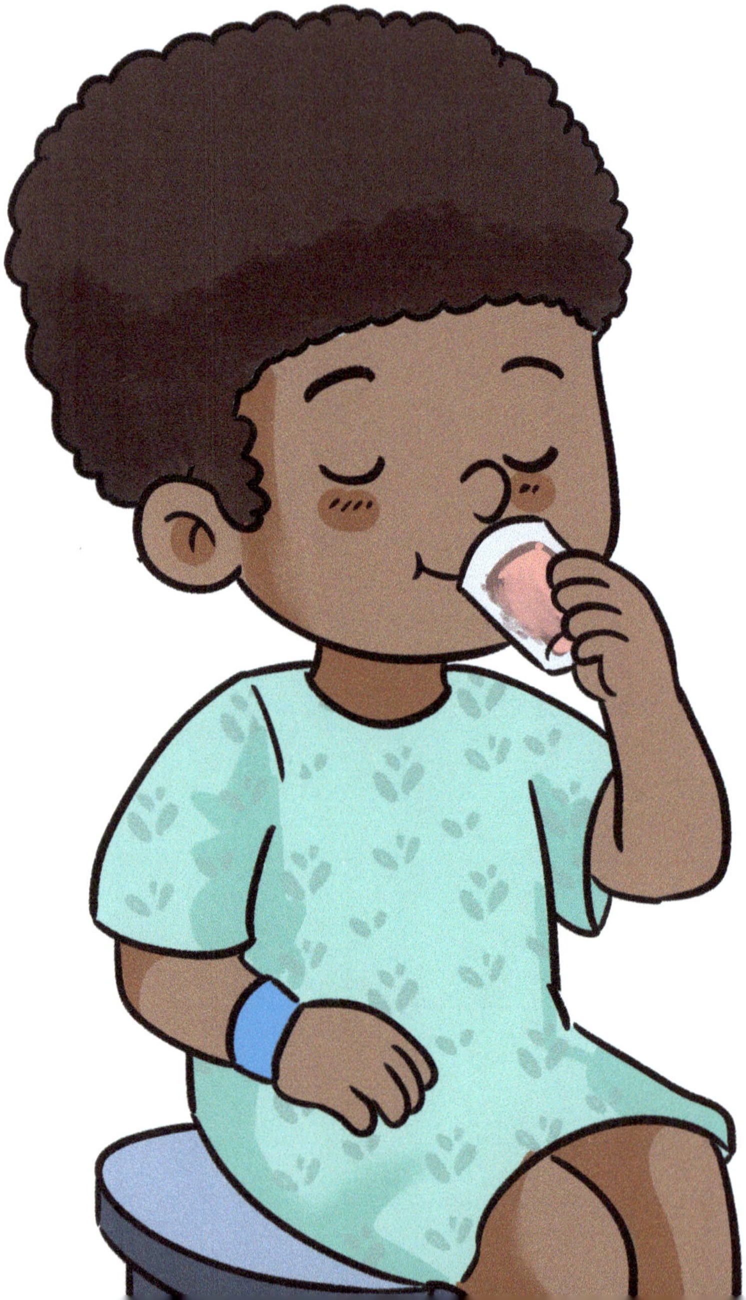

You may need a small IV for your MRI.
An IV is a tiny straw that gives your body medicine.

You might feel a quick poke that lasts just a moment.

Sometimes numbing cream is used to help your skin feel more comfortable.

Other times, the IV is placed after you are asleep.

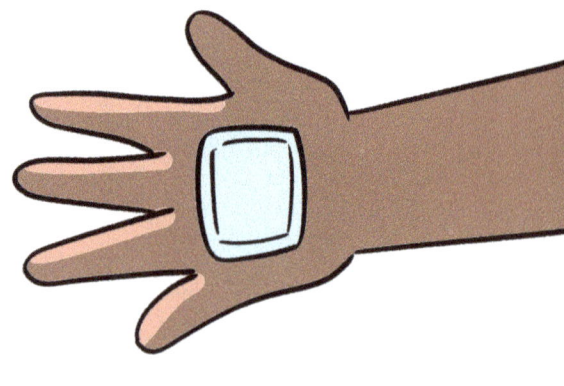

Your doctors and nurses will choose
the safest way to take care of you.

IV catheters come in different colors.

What color will you get? Circle your IV color below.

yellow   blue   pink   green   gray   orange

You've got this!

You and your parent or guardian will meet your medical team before your MRI scan.

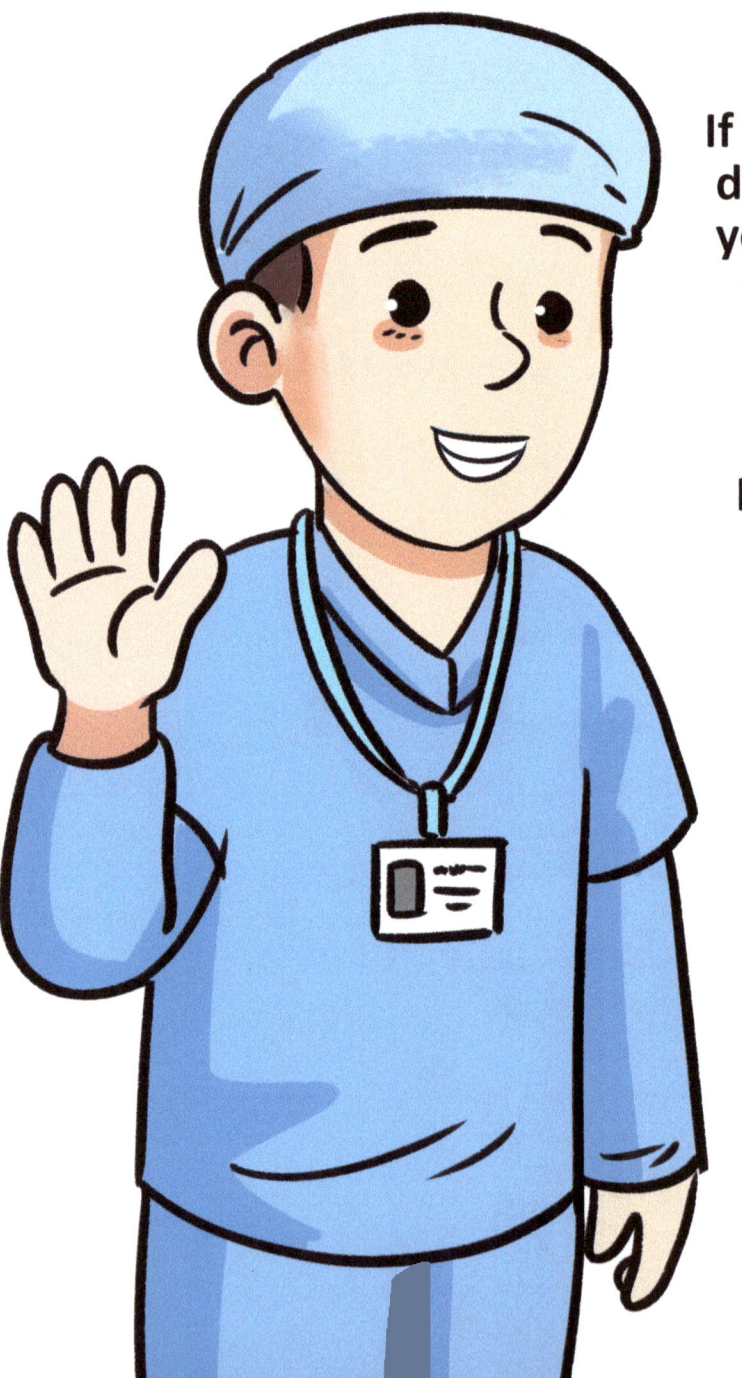

If you are going to take a nap during the scan, you'll meet your anesthesia doctor who is friendly and kind and is happy to answer any questions you may have.

If you have any questions, feel free to ask!

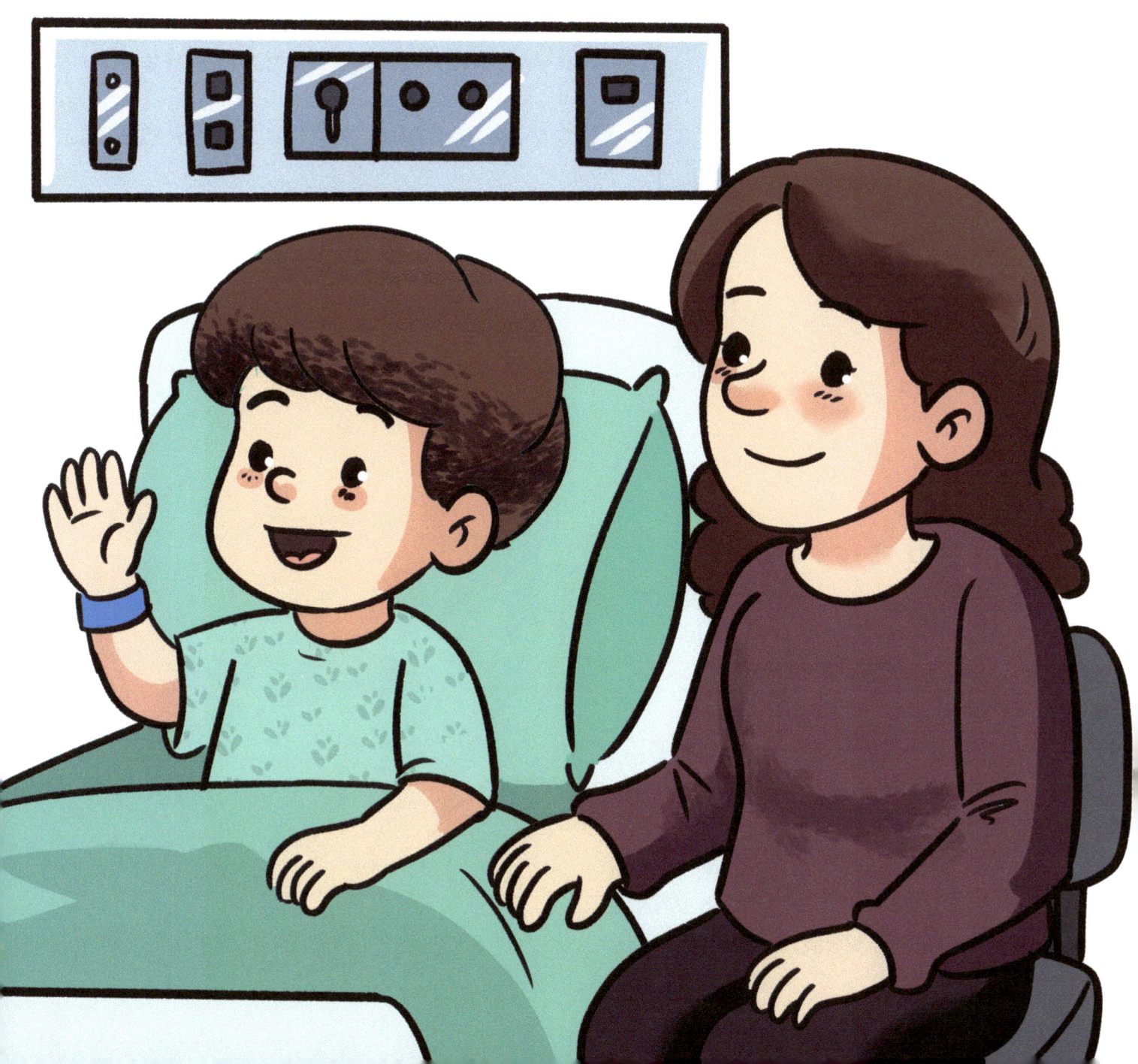

You are strong!

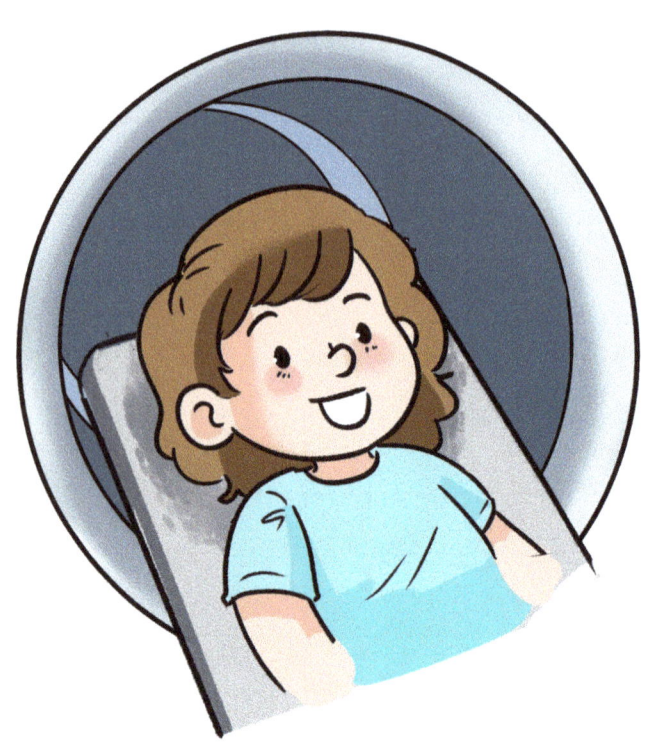

You can stay awake for your special picture time if you can lie very still.

Or you can take a cozy nap instead.

Staying still helps the pictures come out nice and clear.

If you stay awake, try to be as still as a statue — like playing a quiet game of "freeze."

You can keep breathing normally the whole time.

You and your grown-up will decide together what feels best for you.

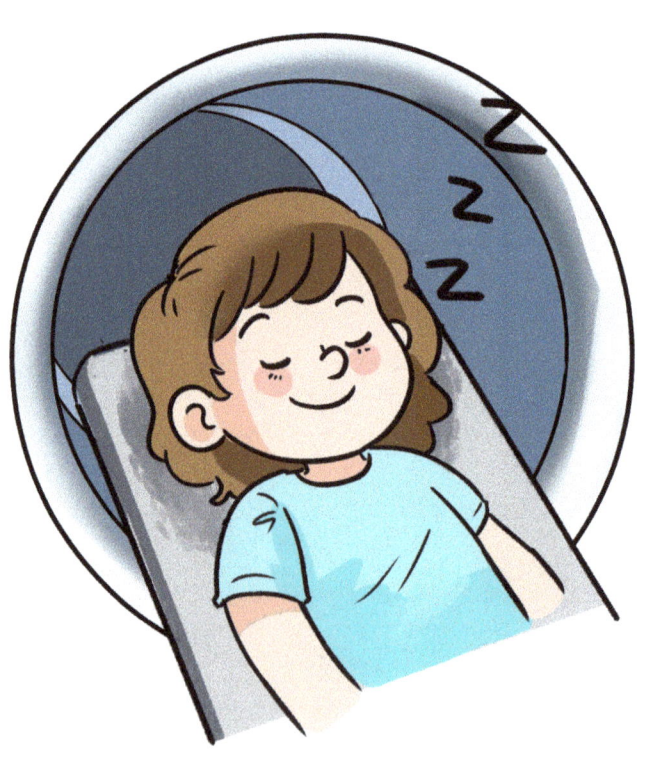

a game of "freeze" | a statue | push button

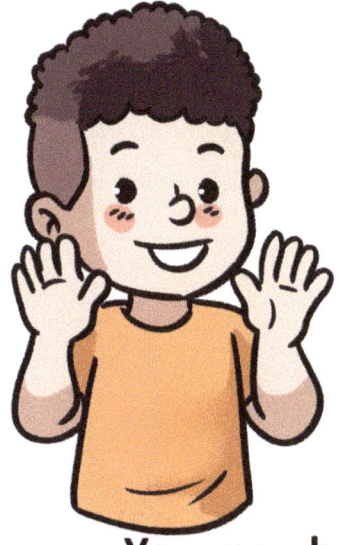
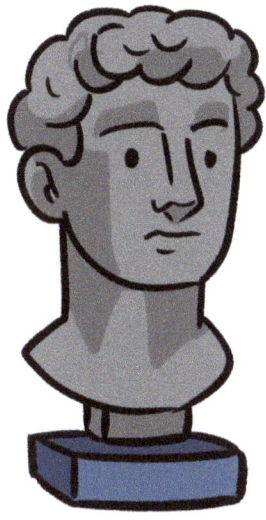
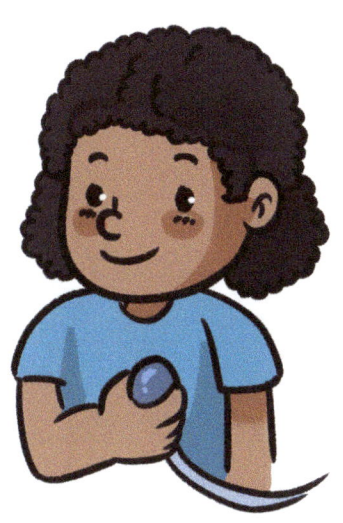

You may be given a button to push if you need to talk to the MRI technician.

What ideas do you have to help you stay still?

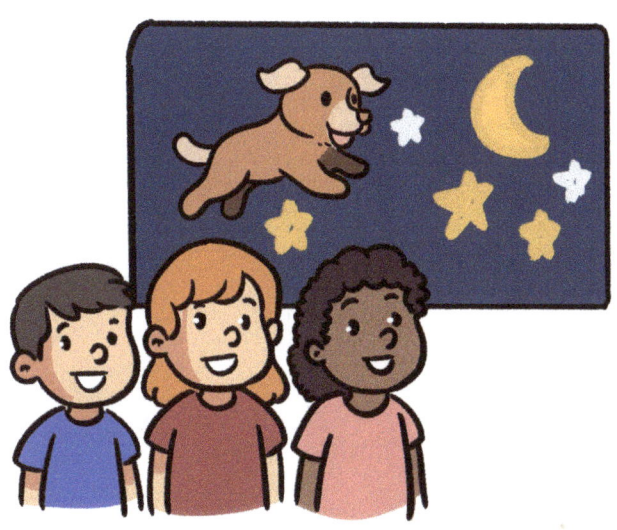
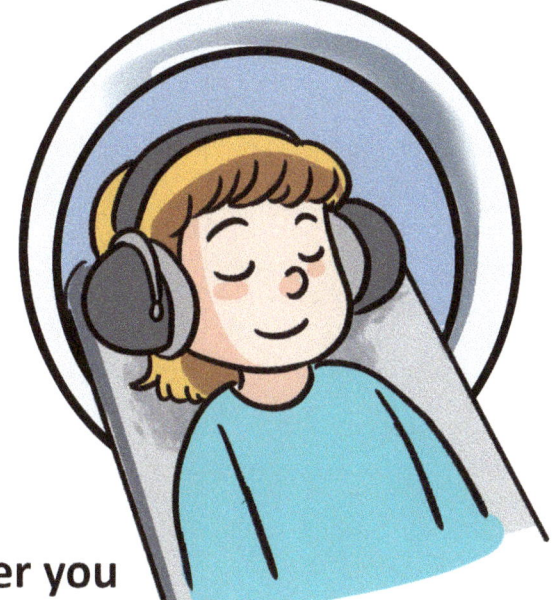

Some MRI scans may be able to offer you a movie to watch or music to listen to while you're getting your pictures taken.

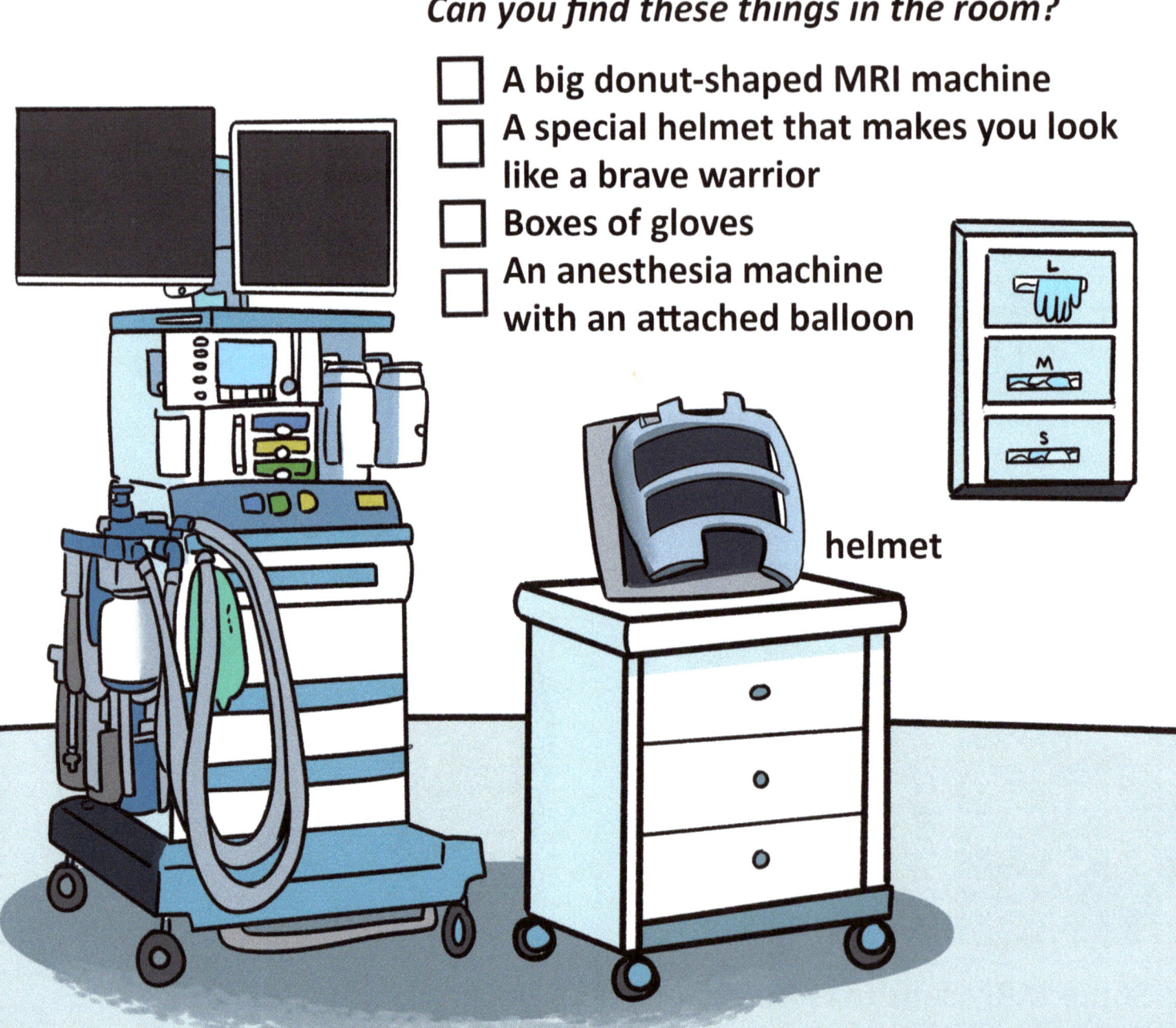

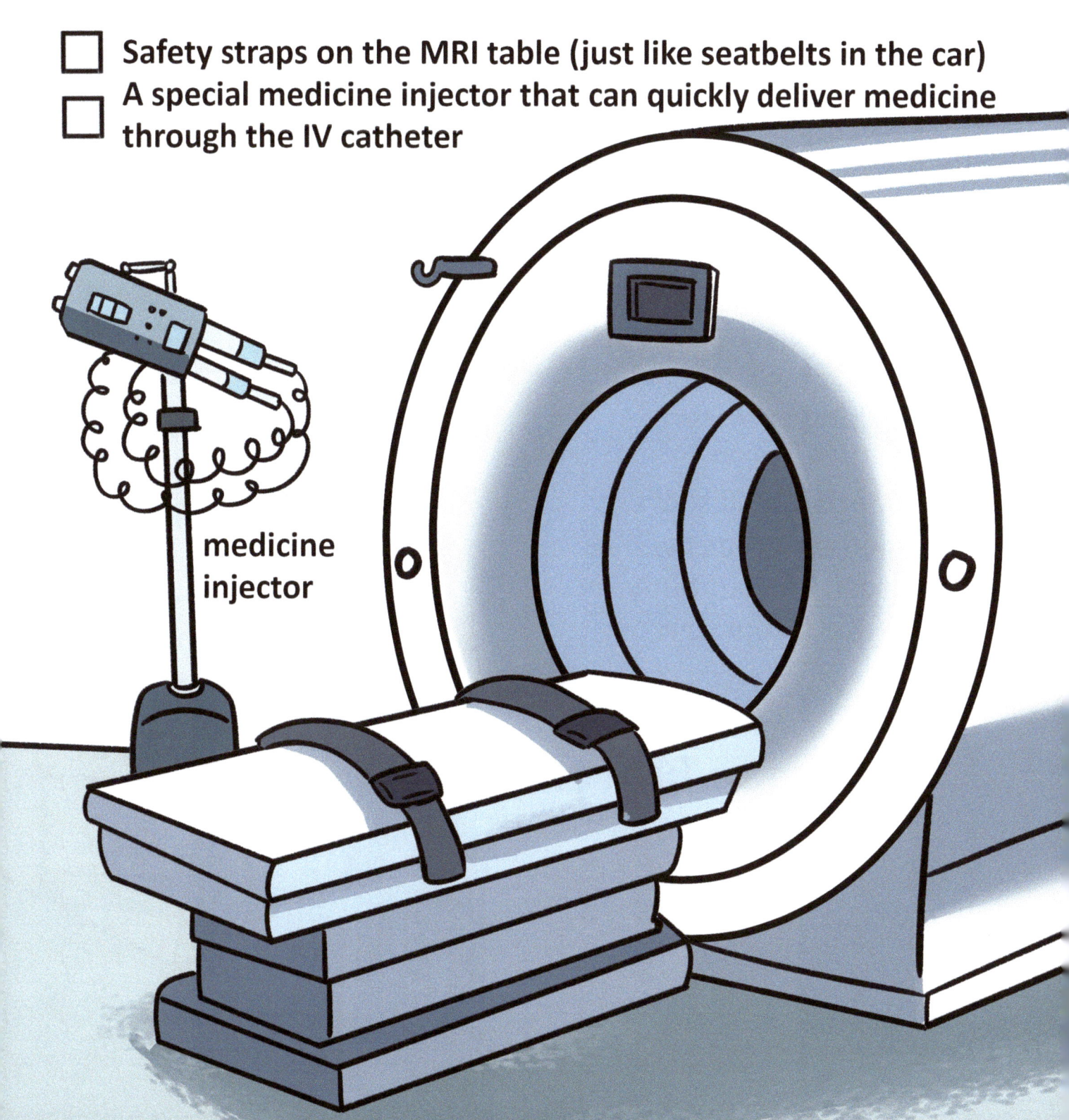

After you get on the bed, they will check your heart, lungs, breathing, and blood pressure.

Special small stickers called electrodes will be placed on your body to check your heart.

You are so brave!

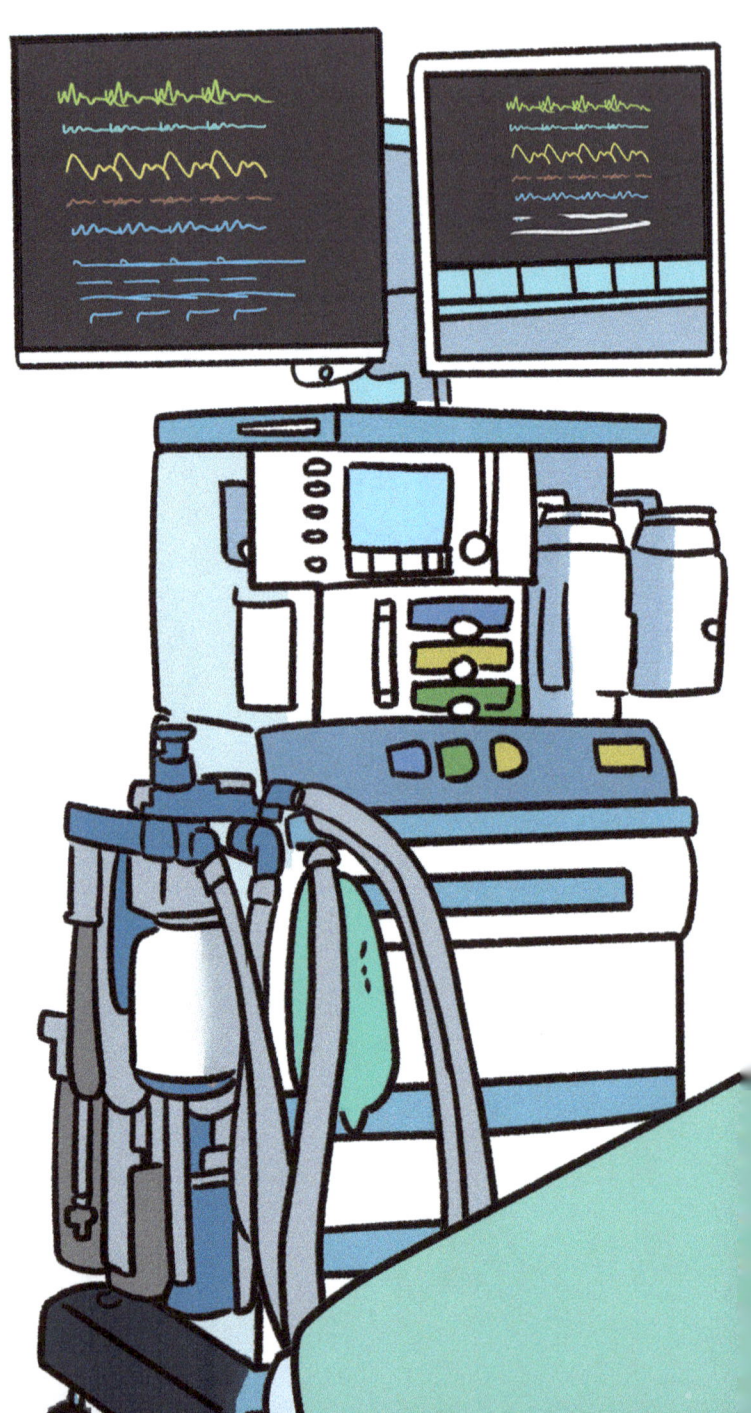

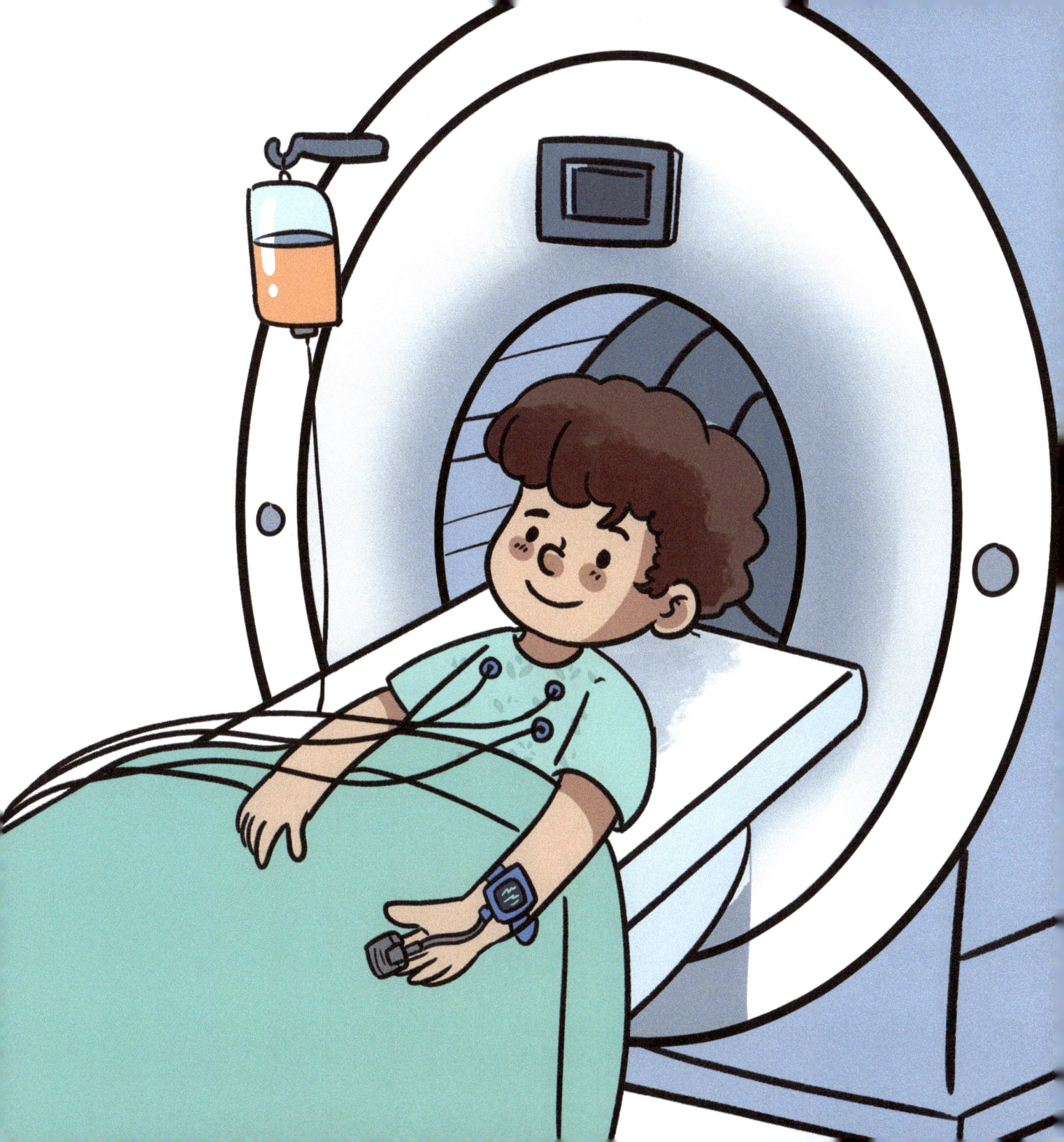

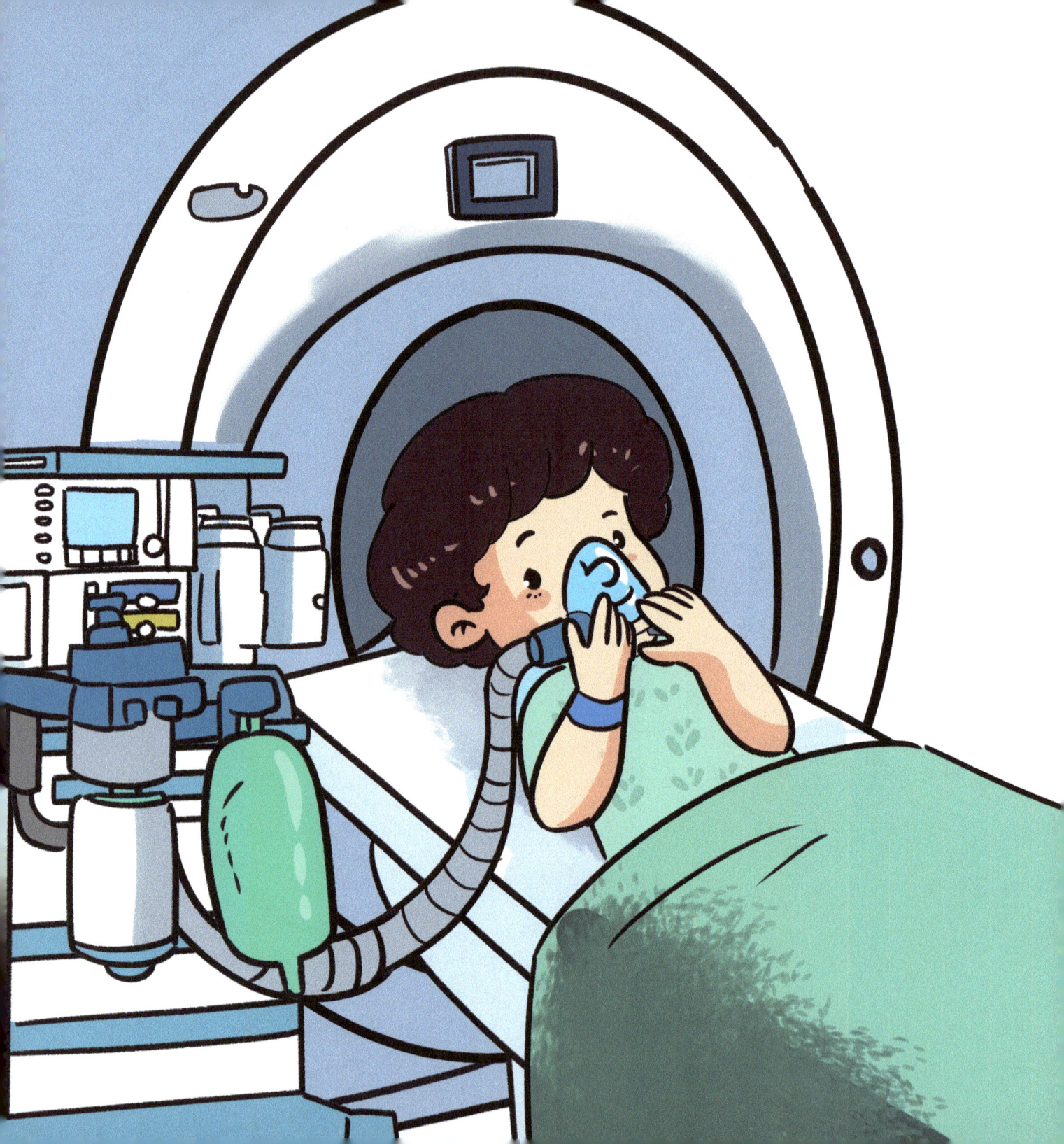

If you're going to sleep, you may get medicine through your IV...

Or you may breathe sleepy air through a soft mask.

Did you know they can make your mask smell sweet and delicious like bubble gum or your favorite fruit?

Draw or write down what scent you would like:

_____

You can see your breathing by looking at the balloon attached to the anesthesia machine.

Cool, right?

Challenge: *Can you blow into your mask and see if you can make the balloon bigger?*

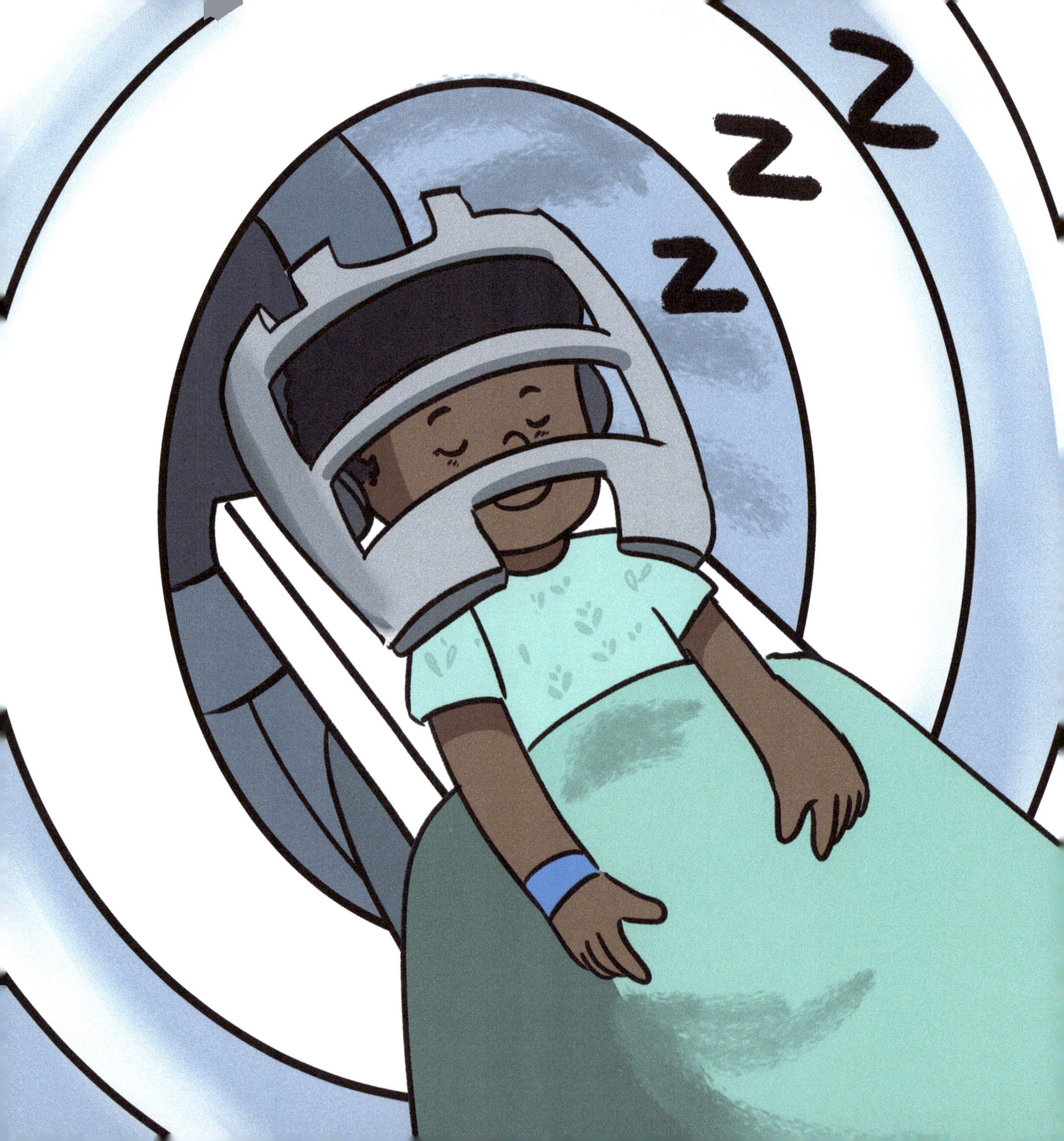

Soon, you will feel sleepy and want to take a nap.

Do you have a nice dream picked out for your nap?

What would you like to dream about?

During your MRI scan, you'll be kept safe and comfortable.

Sweet dreams...

When you wake up from your nap, your MRI scan will be all done.
If you stayed awake during your scan, you can go home right away.

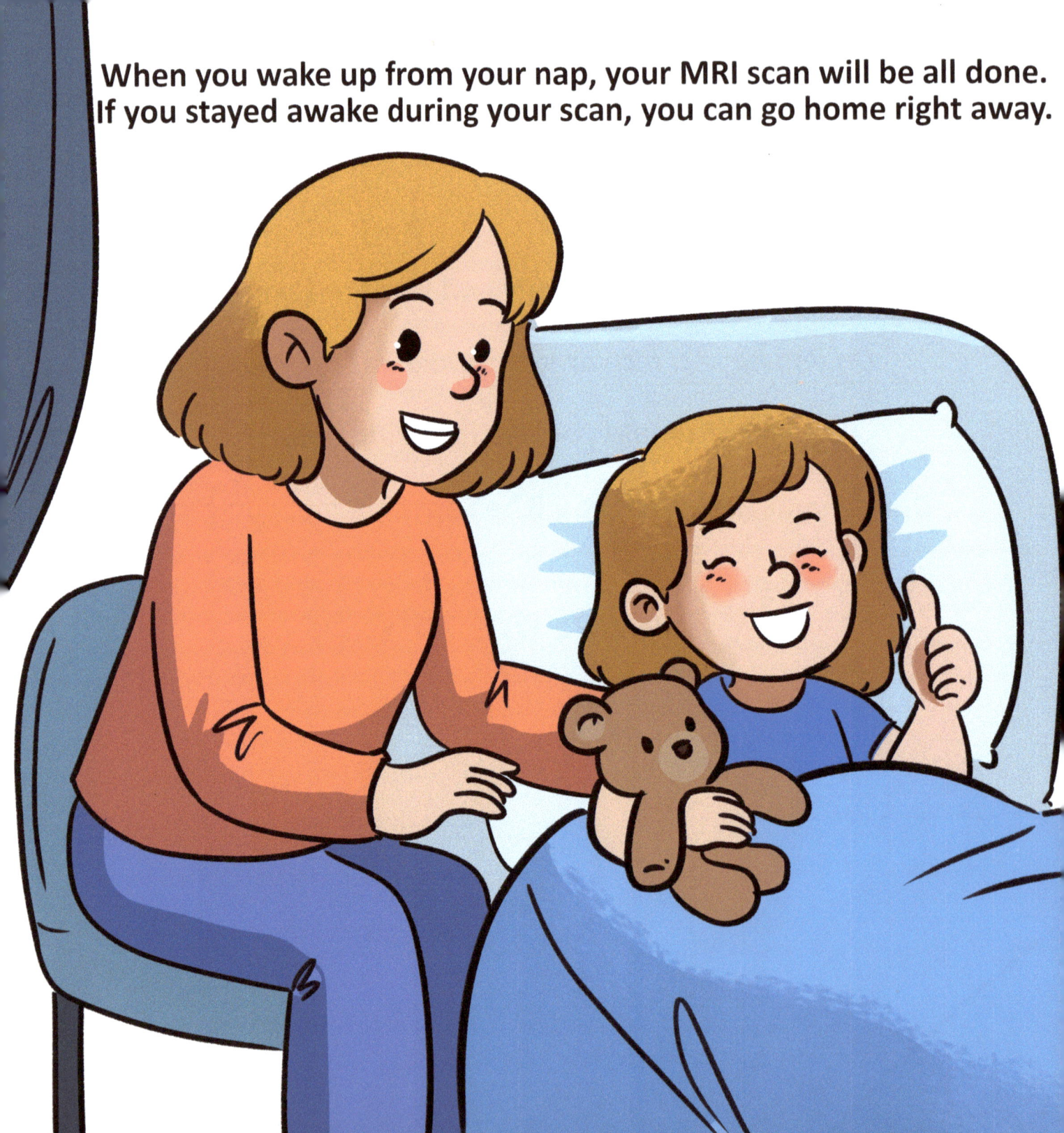

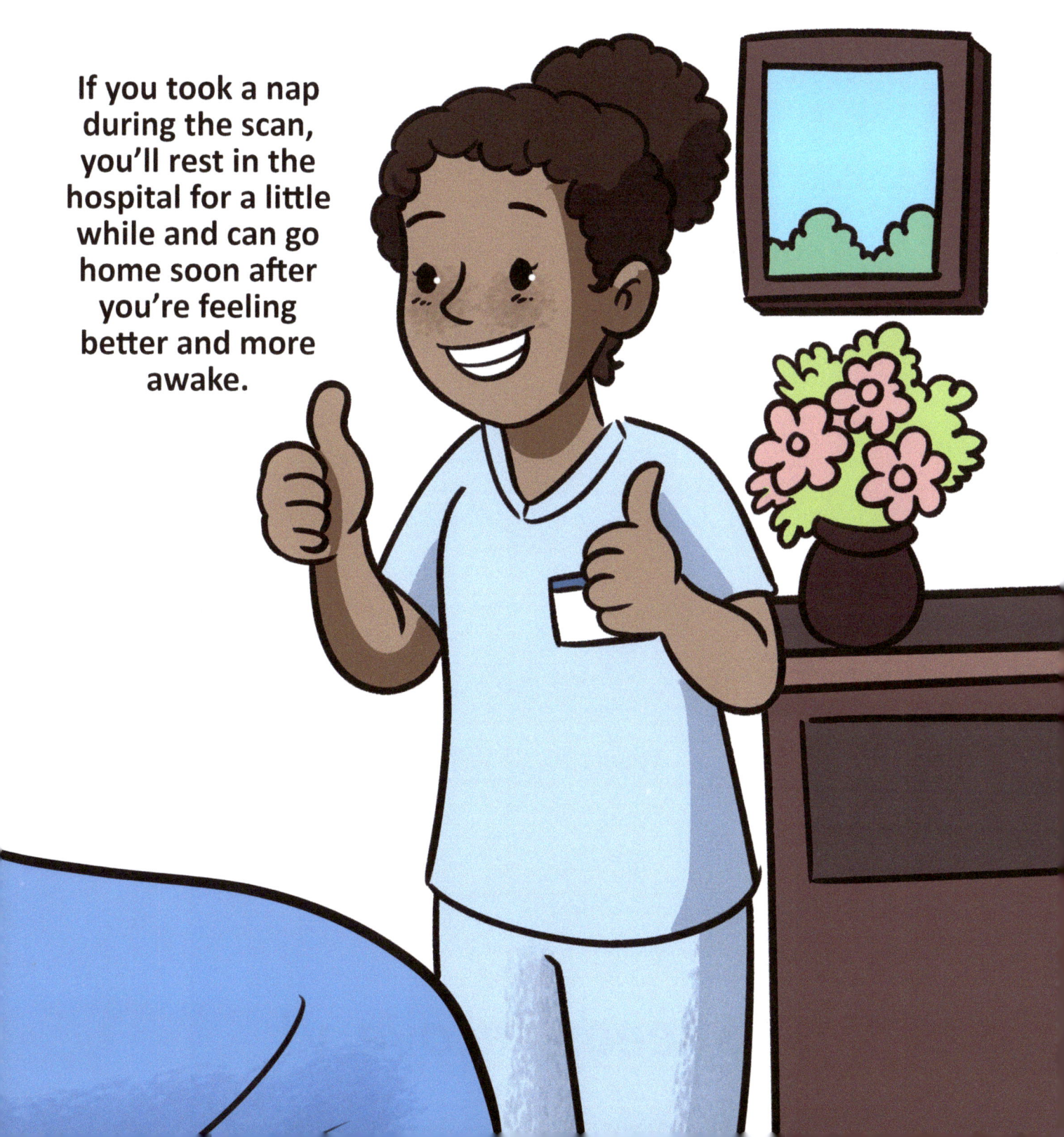

What will you do after your MRI scan?

A party? A celebration?

What's your favorite way to celebrate?

Draw or write your party plan below.

Speedy recovery!

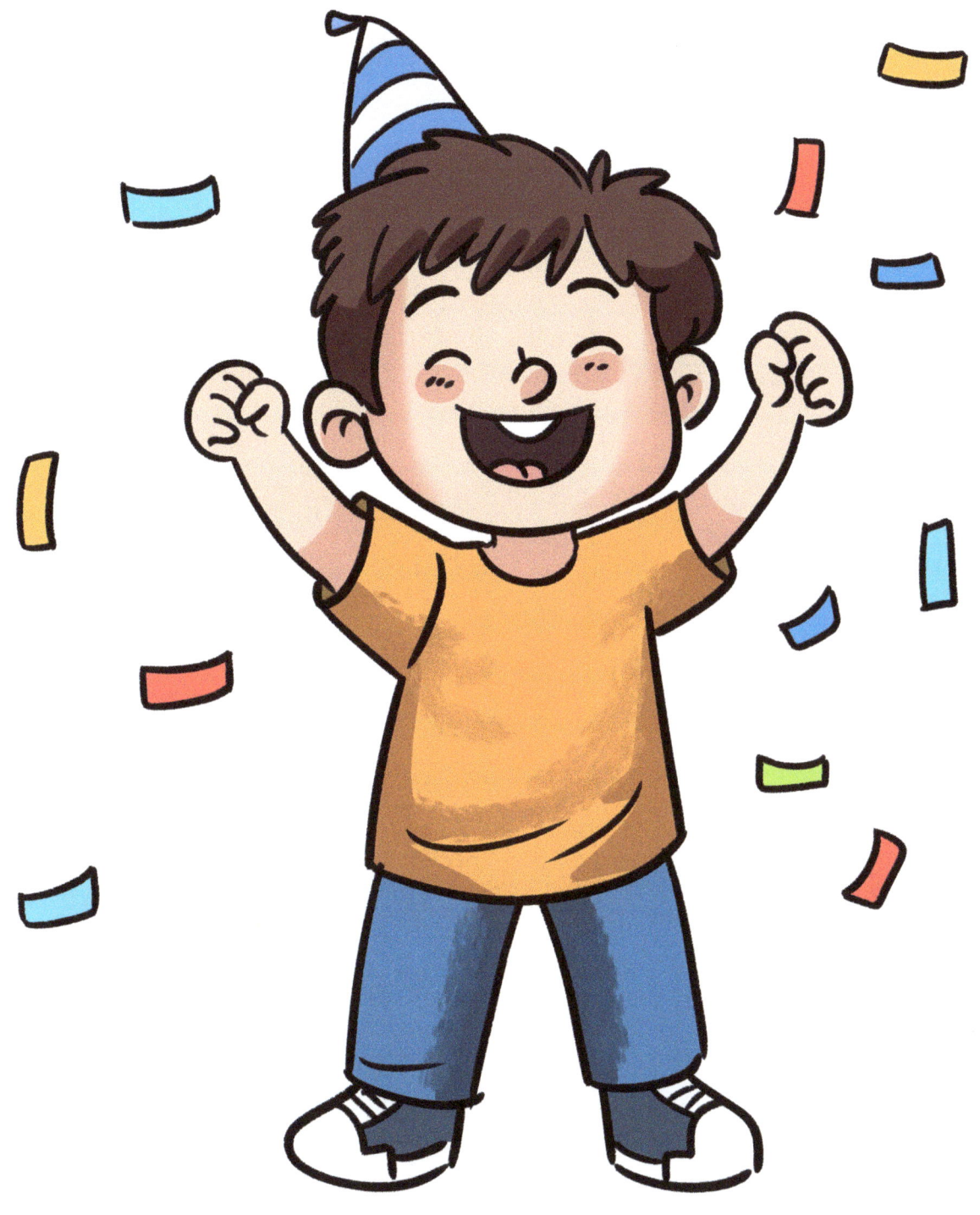

Notes for Parent/Guardian

- If your child stays awake, they can talk with the MRI team through a two-way intercom.

- If your child goes to sleep, the placement of the intravenous (IV) catheter in this young age group can be done after your child is asleep.

- In some cases, contrast medicine may be given through an IV catheter during the MRI scan to help make certain pictures clearer. If contrast is needed, your child may need to have blood work done before the day of the MRI to make sure their kidneys are working well enough to remove the contrast medicine from their body.

- If your child receives anesthesia, it is common for them to feel confused, disoriented, or irritable after the MRI scan. They may cry, sob, kick, scream, or thrash around. It usually takes about one hour for the anesthesia to wear off.

Disclaimer

Please note that the illustrations are not drawn to scale.

This book is written for informational, educational, and personal growth purposes and should not be used as a substitute for medical advice.

Please consult your child's doctor if they need medical attention and to ensure the information in this book pertains to your child's medical condition and needs. I cannot guarantee what your child experiences is exactly what is being discussed in this book.

The author and the publisher are not responsible, either directly or indirectly, for any damages, monetary losses, or reparations due to information in this book. By reading this book, the readers agree not to hold the author and the publisher responsible for any losses as a result of any errors, inaccuracies, or omissions in this book.

Please keep in mind that your child's experience depends on the location, the facility, their medical condition, and the healthcare team.
Please use this book in conjunction with your child's doctor's advice. Thank you.

Did this picture book help your child in some way?
If so, I would love to hear about it!

www.amazon.com/gp/product-review/B0FVWK19ZC

For other book titles, please visit:

www.fzwbooks.com

Connect with the author

email: books@fzwbooks.com
facebook/instagram: @FZWbooks

About the Author

Dr. Fei Zheng-Ward is a clinical anesthesiologist who understands the apprehension patients (both adults and children) may have surrounding their upcoming surgery. Her goal in her medical books is to bring useful information to patients so they have a better understanding and appreciation of what happens leading up to, during, and after surgery. She wants readers to be more empowered to make informed decisions and to feel more at ease with their surgery.

As a practicing physician, she takes pride in being respected for her attention to detail, commitment to providing compassionate and personalized patient care, and strong presence in patient advocacy in the perioperative period for each of her patients. She understands the importance of physical and emotional well-being and advocates for patient autonomy.

Her other children's books aim to bring laughter into your family, encourage children to be more helpful at home, and inspire a love of reading.

She is an award-winning author for her book titled ***What to Expect and How to Prepare for Your Surgery***.

More about Dr. Fei Zheng-Ward:

- Board Certified Anesthesiologist

- Anesthesiology Residency Training at The Johns Hopkins Hospital in Baltimore, MD

- Master in Public Health (MPH) degree from Dartmouth Medical School in Hanover, NH

Books by the author

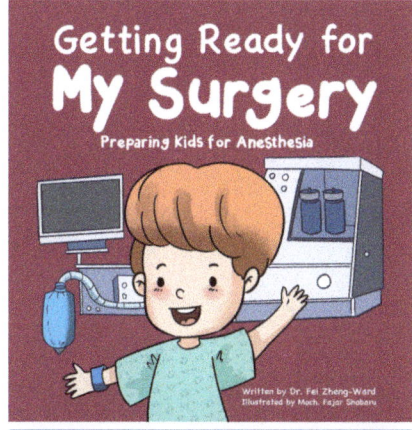
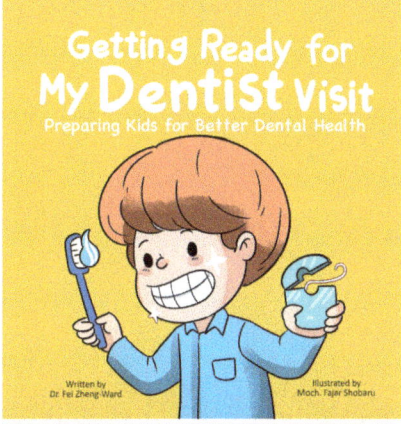
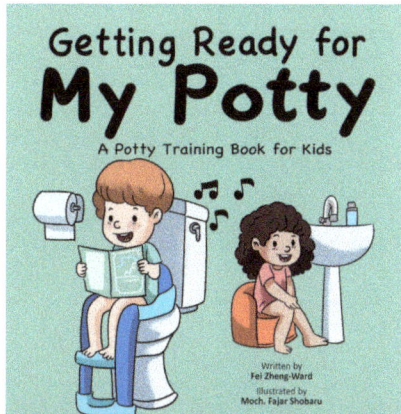
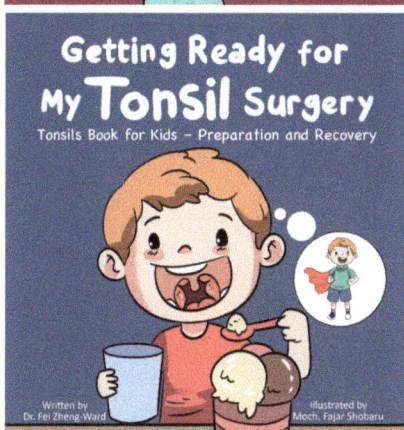
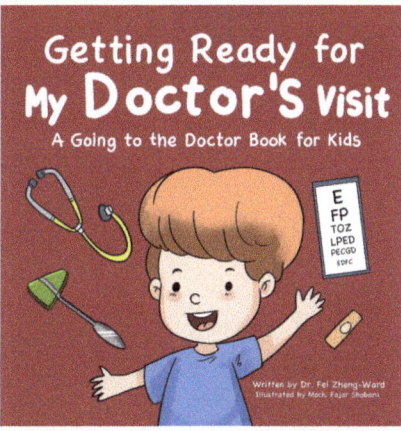
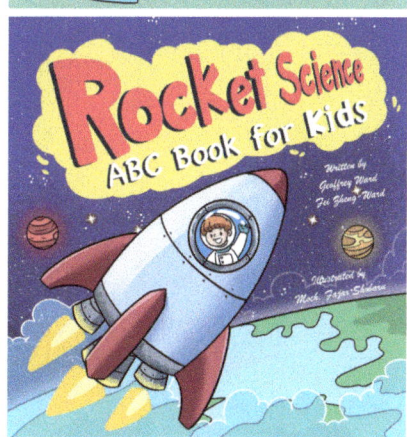
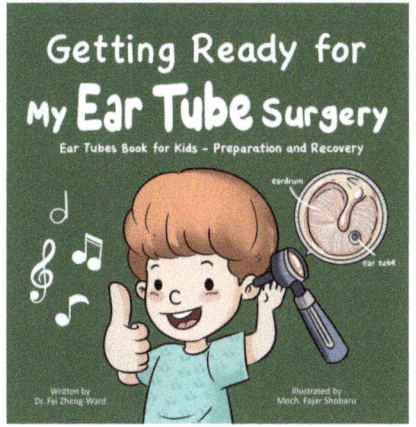
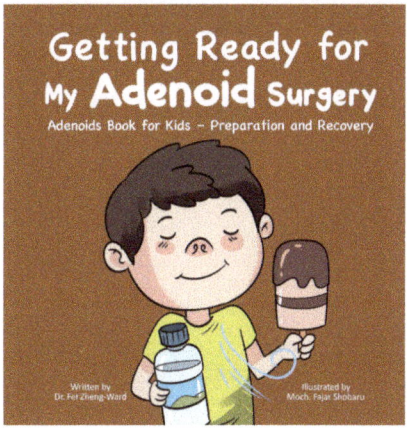
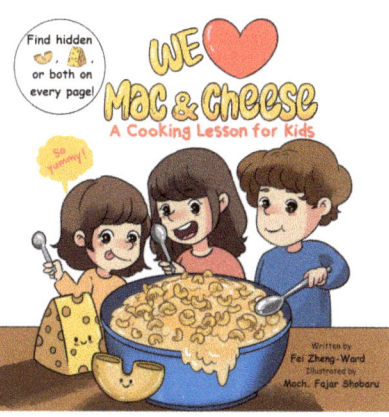

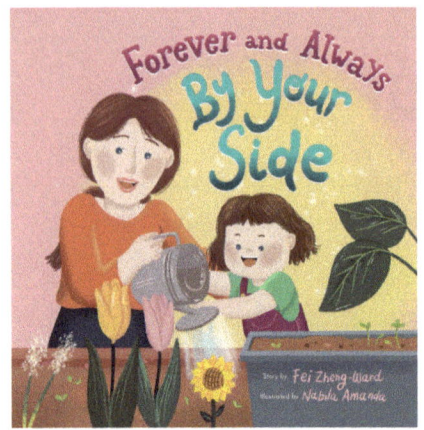
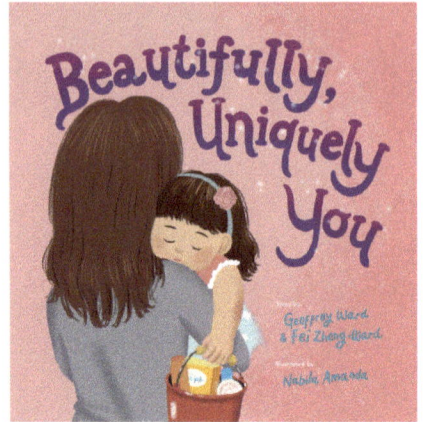
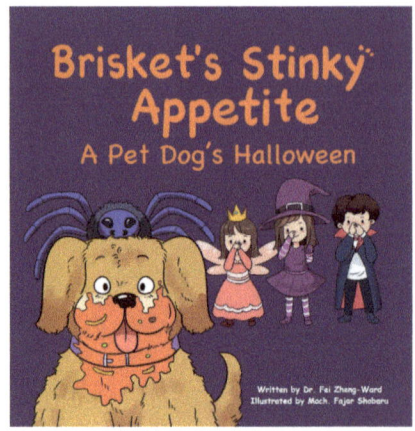
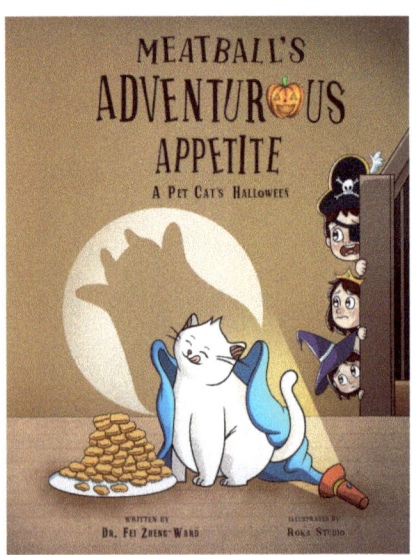
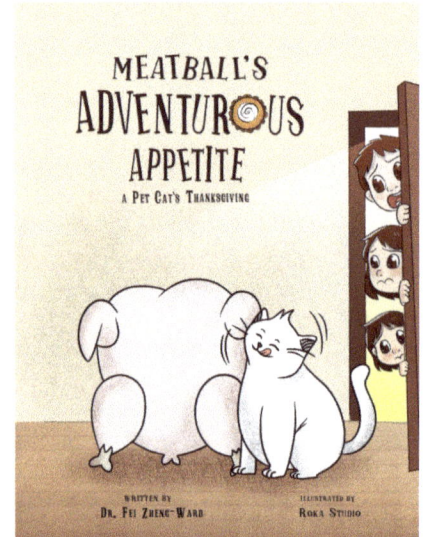
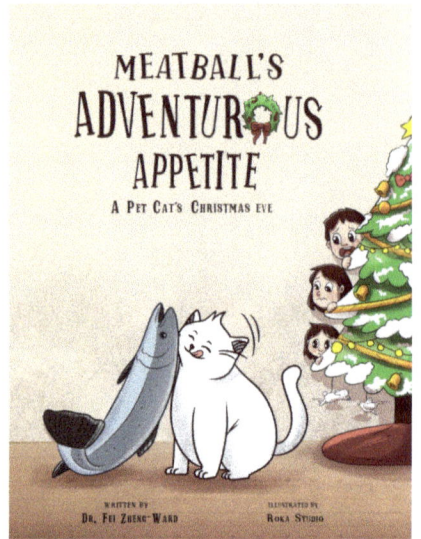
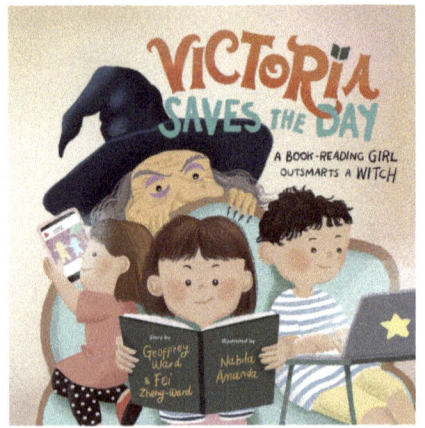
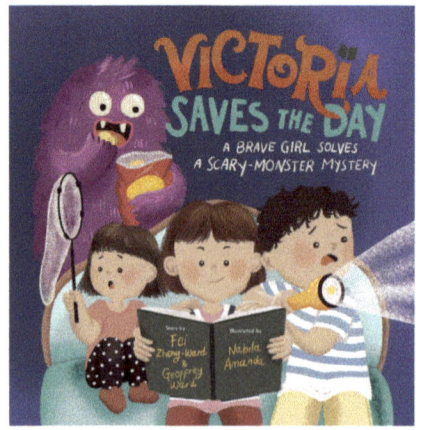
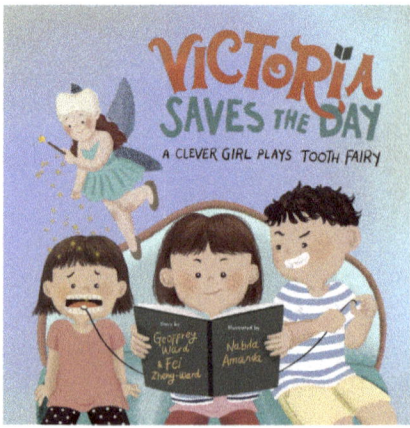

www.ingramcontent.com/pod-product-compliance
Lightning Source LLC
Chambersburg PA
CBHW042359030426
42337CB00032B/5164